Praise for Dr. Laura Liberman's *I Signed as the Doctor*

"A lucid look at cancer when an eminent doctor becomes a patient. Laura Liberman's touching personal and expert professional insights, humanity and down-right helpful advice should be read by those who have cancer and those who treat this disease. Actually, it's a great read for everyone."

> -Barbara Goldsmith, bestselling author and historian,
> Winner of 2007 American Institute of Physics Best Book
> for *Obsessive Genius: The Inner World of Marie Curie*

"When a reader laughs and cries at the same time, that's a sign of a great book. Laura Liberman's true story does it. I love *I Signed as the Doctor*! It made my heart sing."

> -Ellen Daniell, author, *Every Other Thursday: Stories and Strategies from Successful Women Scientists*

"Music and medicine are healing arts. This memoir of a doctor facing her cancer with resilience persuasively describes music's potential for spiritual uplift and for synergy with medicine to heal the body and mind."

> -Richard Kogan, M.D., psychiatrist and concert pianist;
> creator of DVD series, *Music & The Mind*

"Laura Liberman makes the extraordinary possible. The author inspires by her openness and sharing of perspectives. Particularly compelling are her images of family life, reordering priorities, calmness during treatment, and insights into pain control. *I Signed as the Doctor* will help patients cope with illness and will help physicians be better doctors."

> -Kathleen Foley, M.D., neurologist, Pain & Palliative Care
> Service, Memorial Sloan-Kettering Cancer Center

D0725575

I SIGNED AS
THE DOCTOR

Memoir of a Cancer Doctor Surviving Cancer

3/18/09

To Diane –

Best wishes

Paperback:
ISBN-13:   978-0-9822590-0-9
ISBN-10:   0-9822590-0-X

Hardcover:
ISBN-13:   978-0-9822590-1-6
ISBN-10:   0-9822590-1-8

Printed in the United States of America.
Library of Congress Control Number: 2009900330

This book does not provide medical advice such as that obtained in a direct consultation, and does not replace it. No recommendations regarding diagnosis or therapy are being made in this book by the author or by Memorial Sloan-Kettering Cancer Center. Medical issues that concern readers should be addressed directly with their health care practitioners.

About the cover:
The cover photos were taken by master photographer Richard I. DeWitt with permission of milliner extraordinaire Christine A. Moore (http://www.camhats.com/about/html). The front cover photo depicts Laura in Christine's New York studio, trying on hats as she did before beginning chemotherapy.

www.LauraLiberman.com
Booklocker.com, Inc.
2009

I SIGNED AS THE DOCTOR

Memoir of a Cancer Doctor Surviving Cancer

Laura Liberman, M.D.

DEDICATION

This book is dedicated to my husband and the love of my life, David, and to our amazing two children, who make every day joyous. I thank the incredible Jennifer Menell, my "gentle reader," and Cynthia Thornton, my guardian angel. I offer my work to all people living with cancer or other illness (either personally or in a loved one), whether recently diagnosed, in treatment, or survivors. This book is for us.

TABLE OF CONTENTS

FOREWORD

After I had been a radiologist at Memorial Sloan-Kettering Cancer Center in New York for 17 years, I developed left arm numbness, heaviness, and loss of dexterity. I consulted a neurologist and had three months of tests that resulted in the diagnosis of widely disseminated lymphoma, a malignancy of the lymphocytes, which are a group of white blood cells in the body that normally fight infection. I knew from the beginning that I would be treated at Memorial. I worked at the best cancer hospital in the world—where else would I go?

This book is organized primarily as a collection of emails that I wrote immediately before, during, and after treatment. Most of the emails are to my dear friend Jen, although a few are to other people. Occasionally I include an email sent to me by someone else. In writing this book, I aim to tell a survival story accessible to all readers, to help people living with cancer or other serious illness (either personally or in a loved one), and to help doctors take better care of their patients, from my unique perspective as both a cancer doctor and a cancer survivor.

My friends who were kind enough to read and comment on the manuscript have asked me if it is memoir or fiction. The book is memoir. As President Barack Obama writes in the introduction to *Dreams from My Father,* the book is almost entirely true as written, but I have taken liberties, such as altering the order, time frame, or dates of events, compressing two characters into one, and changing some of the characters' names or backgrounds, primarily to protect the privacy of others.

I gratefully acknowledge the help of my friends, including Ellen, who suggested that I write about my cancer experience; Maureen, who used her cancer battle to guide me through mine; my sister-in-law, Laura, whose resilience and humor gave me hope; Monique ("Q"), who helped me believe that I would survive; and Christine, who makes the world's most fabulous hats. I'm indebted to Richard I. Dewitt for magnificent photography, Todd Engel for beautiful cover design, Angela Hoy for shepherding me through the publication process, and Steve Bennett and colleagues at AuthorBytes for spectacular work on the website, www.LauraLiberman.com.

I thank my father for his love and inspiration; his spirit is always with me. I thank my mother for her caring, support, and priceless artistic advice. I gratefully acknowledge my brother for teaching me the alphabet when I was three and for always being able to make me laugh. Thanks to all who wrote to me and prayed for me during my treatment, and to the amazing doctors and nurses at Memorial Sloan-Kettering Cancer Center, who saved my life.

Laura Liberman, M.D.

Chapter 1
Getting Ready

Reach out to your friends. Write about it.

From: Laura
Sent: Friday, March 2, 2007 10:55 PM
To: Jennifer
Subject: News

Hi Jen. I had hoped to talk to you on the phone today, but I'm in a whirlwind. I've just been diagnosed with an aggressive lymphoma, involving lymph nodes, bone marrow, spinal cord, and the fluid around my brain. I have to have a tube put into my chest on Monday, David and I tell the kids next weekend, I get another tube put in my brain the following Monday, and I start chemo on Thurs 3/15.

Apparently I've got a 50/50 shot of going into remission if I do this. I can make a 50/50 shot, don't you think?

I'll be playing stuff by ear—probably not taking care of patients for awhile, but will continue my research and administrative work.

I know that neither of us was religious when you lived in New York City, but we haven't talked about it for awhile. If you pray, please put in a word for me; if you don't, would you mind starting now?

Love
Laura

From: Laura
Sent: Monday, March 5, 2007 9:37 PM
To: Jennifer
Subject: Today

Hi Jen. Today I had a tube called a Mediport catheter put in my chest in Interventional Radiology. Phil, my oncologist, said it wasn't essential—that if I didn't want the catheter, they could just put in an intravenous (IV) every time I need to get IV chemo—but I've seen too many patients who get stuck for every chemo, and they dread it. Also, it sounds like I'll need six months of chemo, a lot of which will be intravenous. There's no way my veins would hold out through all that. I figured getting the catheter would spare my veins from repeated needle sticks. And they said they can take it out after I've finished all of the chemo treatments.

The Mediport was no big deal. They give you IV sedation and then do the procedure under local anesthesia, using fluoroscopy, which looks like a TV screen that shows you x-rays of what's going on in your body, so they can see what they're doing. After making a tiny incision, they insert this sterile plastic catheter into the superior vena cava, a big vein in the chest that leads directly to the heart, and then close the skin over it. They put some sticky stuff called Dermabond on the skin over where the incision was made to help it heal, and then place a bandage over that. Once you have the catheter, they can deliver all the IV chemo through that.

It feels so odd to be a patient at the cancer hospital where I've been a doctor for 17 years. I must have thought that being a doctor, wearing that white coat, confers immunity—like cancer is something that happens to other people, and couldn't

2

possibly happen to me—but apparently that's not the case. When they brought me the consent form for the Mediport, I signed the wrong part—I signed as the doctor, because that's where I always sign! They said no, you have to sign as the patient now. Sometimes I feel like I'm in a play where I know all the lines, but they have me reading the wrong part.

Write to me—little things about you, Sophie, Jim, music, work, life in Philadelphia, and how your pregnancy is going.

Love
Laura

From: Laura
Sent: Tuesday, March 6, 2007 8:10 PM
To: Jennifer
Subject: Chemo

Hi Jen. It's great that you're still finding time to play the cello. I haven't been playing the piano much these days, although I'm a dedicated listener. I miss playing music with you. For me, the best thing about taking that chamber music class at Mannes Conservatory ten years ago was that we got to meet! It was a real departure for me, because in all of my piano training as a kid, my teacher insisted that being a soloist was all that mattered; playing with another person was considered "accompanying" and a lesser art. I'm glad she was wrong.

When we met in that music class, I thought it was so cool that you played the cello, especially since traditionally the cello used to be considered "unladylike." I thought, "Here's a woman unabashed by gender stereotypes." You go, girl.

Let me fill you in on how this all began and what treatment I'm going to get. Around Thanksgiving, I started to have neurological symptoms including loss of fine control in my left arm and left hand. It was subtle—I noticed it most when I was doing breast needle biopsies, because hitting a tiny target requires precise control of both hands, and my left hand just wasn't doing what it was supposed to do. I saw a neurologist at my hospital named Sam, an expert in the field. Sam thought my neuro exam was OK, but he decided to do more tests.

I won't bore you with the details, but the bottom line is that I had magnetic resonance imaging (MRI) exams that showed a mass in the cervical spinal cord, the area in the neck where Christopher Reeve's paralyzing injury was. I had a spinal tap, which they call a lumbar puncture or LP, a procedure in which they stick a needle into your back and take out some fluid from around your spine and brain. I then had surgery to remove an enlarged lymph node. Subsequently, I had a bone marrow biopsy, which must be the most painful procedure on earth. The tests showed lymphoma, a malignancy of lymphocytes, a type of white blood cell that fights infection. Thank God for Sam— he was like a dog with a bone, and he wouldn't let go until he got the diagnosis. Then he referred me to Phil, one of the best lymphoma docs here, to talk about treatment.

My husband came with me to see Phil for that appointment. Phil said it's good that I'm relatively young (47) and pretty healthy, but not good that the lymphoma is in multiple sites (Stage IV), including the central nervous system. He discussed it with the other lymphoma docs, and they want to give me three different kinds of chemo, each one about six times, so probably 18 treatments in all, over the next six months. He says that even one of these kinds of chemo is tough to tolerate; three will be a real challenge.

For the lymph nodes and bone marrow, I need IV chemo called R-CHOP. The R is Rituximab, a monoclonal antibody directed against the specific malignant cells in my lymphoma; C is cyclophosphamide (also called cytoxan); H is doxorubicin (formerly Adriamycin; don't ask me why they use "H" for that); O is vincristine (originally called Oncovin, hence the O); and P is prednisone, an oral steroid. The R-CHOP will be given at least once a month for six months; I go to the outpatient chemo suite, get my Mediport hooked up to an IV, and stay for seven or eight hours; then I go home on five days of oral prednisone.

The second kind of chemo is called high-dose IV methotrexate, which I'll also probably need once a month for six months. They need very high doses of methotrexate to get into the spinal cord, and with it they have to give tons of IV fluids because otherwise the methotrexate can crystallize in the kidneys and cause kidney damage. So every time I get it, I have to get admitted to the hospital, have the IV hooked up to my Mediport, get a ton of fluid and the methotrexate, and follow it up with what's called "leukovorin rescue," which helps fight the toxicity of the methotrexate, and I get more fluid to flush the excess methotrexate out of my system. Each admission will be from three to five days.

I also need to get outpatient methotrexate given "intrathecally," which means directly injected into a tube or catheter called an "Omaya" that they are going to neurosurgically implant into my brain. I'll probably need six of those too, but I'm not sure exactly when and how often. Tomorrow, I have an appointment with the neurosurgeon who will put in the Omaya next week, so I'll find out more.

David and I are trying to take all this in as the lymphoma doc is talking. I'm thinking if I'm going to die anyway, maybe I'd rather spend the next few months at home instead of getting brain surgery and chemotherapy. I asked Phil what was the chance of cure. "Cure?" he asked in a tone that suggested that the idea of cure was ludicrous. He said he couldn't cure me, but there's about a 50% chance that he could bring the lymphoma into remission, which means at least temporarily under control. That means that there's a 50% chance that he won't get me into remission and I'll die. Then David and I went to see Sam. I asked Sam if he thought I should get treated, and he said yes.

After we finished with the doctors, David and I went to get a cup of coffee and talk. We were both shell-shocked. "If this is a nightmare, can I wake up now?" I asked him. He paused, head down, before responding, "I wish we could." He looked as scared as I felt, and he doesn't scare easily. I brought up the possibility of declining treatment. My symptoms are mild, I said; maybe the lymphoma will never progress; the treatment may be more dangerous than the disease. I don't want a pyrrhic victory, winning the battle but losing the war—if killing the cancer kills the patient, it doesn't do much good for anybody. But both Phil and Sam think I should be treated, I have a husband and two kids, and I have a 50% chance of surviving. I have to take that chance. I told David I'd take care of the lymphoma if he'd handle the paperwork. Together we'd decide what and how to tell the kids. He nodded.

Jen, I'm scared. I understand all of this stuff intellectually but it's different when you're the one going through it. You can get heart damage from the doxorubicin, permanent neurological changes from the vincristine, manic from the prednisone, and painful ulcers in the lining of your gut anywhere from top to bottom from the IV methotrexate. You can become a vegetable from the brain surgery or from the lymphoma in the central nervous system, and God knows what injecting chemo directly into the fluid around your brain can do. And chemo suppresses your immune system, leaving you vulnerable to infections which can kill you. So you can die from the chemo or from the lymphoma itself.

It's weird. As a doctor, I've always advised patients not to think too far down the line, worrying about stuff that's five steps away, because in medicine, each outcome affects what decisions you'll have to make in the next step. It's best just to deal with the immediate decision, see what happens, and take it from there. Apparently that's easier said than done. Physician, heal thyself.

Please keep writing and praying, and I'll do the same.

Love
Laura

***

From: Laura
Sent: Wednesday, March 7, 2007 9:12 AM
To: Ellen
Subject: Your talk

Hi Ellen. Hope you had a safe trip home!

The talk you gave to our women faculty about your book, *Every Other Thursday*, was incredibly well received. People were inspired by your experience of creating a group for mutual support and guidance consisting of women scientists and administrators that has met every other Thursday for 30 years. I'll send you separately our survey results from your talk; these are among the best scores any event has received in the 15 months the Program for Women Faculty Affairs has existed!

Unfortunately, "Every Other Thursday" now has new meaning for me. I just found out that I have lymphoma, and I gather that my chance of surviving this is 50/50. Next week I begin six months of chemo, which will probably be every two weeks, and usually it will start Thursday: every other Thursday.

My husband has been amazing, and I've also found a small group of close women friends, one of whom has had cancer, who I know will help me get through this. Did your group ever get into health issues? Do you have any suggestions about group work for this?

Best wishes
Laura

From: Ellen
Sent: Wednesday, March 7, 2007 10:03 PM
To: Laura
Subject: Re: Your talk

Dear Laura,

Thank you for the wonderful personal comments and feed-back. I have been telling everyone that the MSKCC talk (and visit) was one of the most interactive and interesting, and just plain FUN that I've had. I'm delighted people responded so positively. Now to move to your personal news.

I am speechless. I received your message this morning from my step-daughter's home, where we often spend Sundays and Mondays; we went directly there from the Oakland airport Sunday when I returned from my east coast visit. I was online because I was checking flights to Florida for a sudden trip: my husband's brother passed away yesterday. It was hard, especially in that context, to process your bad news, but now home, I've reread it several times and settle down to reply. I

8

realize you must have known most of this when we met last week, and understand your choice not to share it and have it "color" our whole interaction, though I would have been glad to talk of it then too. I appreciate your telling me now, and I hope I can be, albeit at a distance, one of the women friends who help you through this. I did feel a strong rapport, over books to be sure, but also attitude! You are perfect for the job you are putting so much into along side your medical profession.

50/50 must be incredibly hard to hear. It is nearly impossible to process statistics of that nature, even (or maybe especially) when your professional life is involved with detection and diagnosis.

Yes, we talk about health issues in Group. Scares that turn out OK (lumps that are benign), and Christine's that was major breast cancer. One of the things I quote in the book from her is "There is a new personal reality that comes from having cancer. When someone says you have a 30 percent instead of 20 percent chance of metastasis, what does that mean in life terms? Do you do something differently?" I remember how we celebrated when she was told chemo wouldn't be necessary, then the doctors reversed that decision based on a cellular observation that none of us really understood in medical terms. I think the MOST important lesson is the value of reaching out, leaning on others whenever you can, and knowing that no matter how supportive and wonderful your family (I'm glad your husband is amazing; he'll need to be, and you deserve it), you need others as well, because your family will be scared along with you.

I feel you know so much more than I do about cancer and medicine, and I'm no guru, even if you do like my book so much. But I will say that talking through the fears, and asking for everything you need and depending on your friends to say when they can't deliver and you need to ask someone else. The ability to ask is all critical. Also, one anecdote (I know everyone has them, but this one is very close to me). My closest friend from college had breast cancer which spread to her brain (10 years after the first diagnosis, lump removal chemo, and radiation, one year after a recurrence and mastectomy). She was given "2-3 years to live" after aggressive radiation. One of the things she chose to do with her time was to visit Peru (Machu Pichu in particular), which she did with a sister, a niece, and me. It was an incredible trip for all of us. But the important thing is that now, six years later, she is still alive, is working (she's a teacher) again, has moved to Oregon where her husband had always wanted to live, and is, well, living. Scans are now every six months instead of every three. Her chances for remission were considered much less than 50/50.

There is a certain fear in writing to someone dealing with such big issues, that one will say something "wrong." Telling you Ruth's story is one of those, and I went back and rewrote it. But I believe that you can sort out the helpful from the useless and will forgive statements that are clumsy or ill-considered. I'll certainly keep in touch, and I ask you to keep me posted as you can. One thing my friend Ruth (above) did was to have a kind of e-mail "cancer journal" that she sent to about 30 friends and relatives that she wanted to keep informed. Sometimes frequent, sometimes with gaps of several months, but a way to share her experience without writing individual letters when her strength was limited.

I am missing yet another Group because of this funeral, but I will some time ask them for advice about group work, especially Christine. And with your permission, I'll tell Ruth about you. She's been involved for years (since way before the cancer) with something called co-counseling and I know that she derived much support from discussions in that structure. But maybe right now is the time for just getting started, and for collecting resources and surrounding yourself with people who can help.

With great affection and all the hope and strength I can offer, Ellen

---

From: Laura
Sent: Thursday, March 8, 2007 5:40 AM
To: Ellen
Subject: Writing

Hi Ellen. Thanks for your speedy response! I love your idea of the "cancer journal." I've been thinking about writing a book about being a cancer patient and a cancer doctor—I think it would help me deal with the experience and might be useful to other cancer patients, their families and friends, and doctors. And yes, please tell Ruth about me. I would love to hear from her and others in your Group.

While you were here, you asked about the other work I do at Memorial, but then we didn't have time to get into it. I came to Memorial as a radiologist specializing in Breast Imaging in 1990, right after I finished training. For the next 15 years, I read mammograms, breast ultrasound exams, and MRI of the breast, and performed breast needle biopsies, where we take a sample of a breast abnormality with a needle to send to pathologists who see whether it's cancer. I teach medical students, residents, fellows, and other doctors. I also do breast cancer research focusing on breast needle biopsies. I've written about 100 scientific papers and co-authored a book—like you, I love to write!

A few years ago, I was a member of a Women's Task Force created by our Physician-in-Chief to discuss issues related to women faculty at Memorial. We had monthly discussions and gave a survey to women faculty to find out their concerns. We found that women were significantly more likely than men to say that they were unclear about promotion criteria, that they lacked a mentor or had a mentor who hindered their career, and that they struggled with issues of work/life balance. We suggested creating an ongoing office to address women faculty issues. The Program for Women Faculty Affairs (PWFA) was created in October 2005, and I was chosen to be the Director.

For the past two years, I've spent two days a week in the Women's Office and three days a week in Breast Imaging. I love my work in the Women's Office. Since the program was new, I got to help create it. I made a database of all faculty that included their departments, ranks, and tracks so I could get baseline data on positions of female vs. male faculty, created a website to share information relevant to women faculty, organized seminars on promotion criteria and other topics of interest to women faculty, began helping women individually with career decisions and promotion packages, and created Athena, an informal networking group for women faculty that meets monthly.

With this illness, I'm especially glad about my mid-career shift. I had reached a point in my life when I want to be more of a mentor and help other women succeed, rather than pursuing the spotlight for myself—kind of like I'd rather play chamber music than be the soloist. The Women's Office work is rewarding but not as physically and emotionally grueling as clinical care of cancer patients. I also have more control over my schedule in the Women's Office than in clinical work. The flexibility will be essential when I'm going through cancer treatment.

Got to go. I don't sleep too well these days. I get up in the middle of the night and read or listen to music for awhile, but then I seem to hit a point when I run out of steam and have to lie down. I just hit that point.

I'll keep you posted. I so appreciate your offer to be one of my women friends who gets me through this!

Warmly
Laura

From: Laura
Sent: Thursday, March 8, 2007 10:07 AM
To: David
Subject: Yes we will

Hi Babe. I love you. We will get through this, and then, what a book I'll have to write!

Love
Laura

Chapter 2
Telling the Kids

Be sensitive to your family.

From: Laura
Sent: Saturday, March 10, 2007 6:43 AM
To: Jennifer
Subject: Saturday

Dearest Jen,

Thank you so much for your daily notes; I can't tell you how much I enjoy reading them. I'm so glad you kept the maternity clothes from your last pregnancy. I bet you look great in your new Pashmina. I've never seen a Pashmina in real life—only on one episode of Friends, when Jennifer Aniston goes out on a shopping spree.

I've been in a flurry of activity since I last wrote. Wednesday I saw the neurosurgeon, Mark, to plan the Omaya. He explained how he was going to neurosurgically insert the Omaya catheter into my brain, so they can deliver chemo directly into the cerebrospinal fluid (CSF), which is the fluid around the brain, around the spinal cord, and in several little water-balloon-like structures in the brain called "ventricles." Mark is a fabulous surgeon and a likeable guy, quiet with a warm sense of humor, although I told him I preferred our relationship when it was limited to my reading films about the hardware he's putting in *other* people! He says they used to do about 50 Omayas a year at Memorial, but now they do about 20. He's done a lot of them, and knows what he's doing.

There were two moments in the visit that I didn't like. The first was when he told me how they have to drill a hole in the skull and put the Omaya through the hole and through brain tissue until the tip reaches one of the ventricles. In describing the procedure, he showed me a picture of a brain with a catheter in it. I had never quite realized how far the ventricles are from the surface of the brain!

The second part of the visit that I didn't like was when he told me the Omaya will be there forever. I hadn't realized that. It makes me feel like my life is divided into my world before this Monday (pre-Omaya) and my world after this Monday (post-Omaya). They also have to do this under general anesthesia. So the brain surgery part is intimidating. You know how in your whole life, when people ask you to do something hard, you always think to yourself, "Well, at least it's not brain surgery!" Well, now it IS brain surgery, so what am I supposed to say—maybe, "It isn't rocket science"?

When the neurosurgeon left the room I asked his nurse who's been at Memorial for 36 years if it was OK to cry for a minute and she said it was. She told me that when she used to be a floor nurse, she would tell the patients they were allowed to cry for 20 minutes a day. Apparently there are no restrictions on the time of day you can cry, and you're able to do it all at once or break it into smaller sessions, eg 2 crying sessions of 10 minutes each, or 4 crying sessions of 5 minutes each, or even 10 crying sessions of 2 minutes each. I took her card and her number. That advice may come in handy.

Wednesday night I dragged David to a seminar run by Social Work on how to tell your kids that you have cancer. I wish you had been there to give me the child psychologist's perspective on the seminar. We met in a small conference room in the hospital. There are three big windows that look out on the Rockefeller campus across the street, but the curtains were drawn. Usually the room is arranged formally, with all the chairs lined up in rows facing the podium in front. For this seminar, it was more casual, with the chairs in a little circle.

David was on my left, and my friend Maureen was on my right. Maureen is a doctor here—last year, when her daughter Julie was 10, Maureen was diagnosed with endometrial cancer, and had surgery, radiation, and chemotherapy. She lost her hair with the chemo, and it's coming back even a more flaming red than it was before. Maureen is heroic and blunt—the cancer was no match for her. She's seen it all, tells it like it is, and is fearless—a terrific ally to have in your corner.

The seminar began by us going around the circle and all the participants introducing themselves and telling why they were there. The people at the seminar were a bizarre mix. The first woman on David's left was an inpatient wearing her hospital gown and pushing her IV pole, and she seemed disturbed. She has cancer widely spread throughout her body, but they aren't sure where it began. Her kids are grown up but she has a 5-year-old granddaughter in her care. She would not stop talking. The social worker finally had to interrupt after she had spent ten minutes on an intensive discussion of every symptom and test she had that led up to her diagnosis of cancer.

On her left was a couple, a man and his extremely pregnant wife, and she was crying hysterically from the moment they walked into the room. I thought she must have something terrible. Turns out her father has cancer, and what they're worried about is, how do they tell their 2-year-old daughter that Grampa is sick? I'm sorry, let's not compete over whose problem is worse, but telling the two-year-old that Grampa is sick just isn't on the same page as telling your teenage kids that you have cancer. Afterwards, Maureen told me, "I know how they should tell their two-year-old. Say 'Grampa's sick,' and then turn on Blue's Clues, and she'll be fine."

The third couple in the group was a husband and wife in their late 30s or early 40s. The mom, who is fine, lost her mother to cancer at a young age, and hadn't been given complete information. The dad has had adrenocortical carcinoma for three years, very aggressive and not treatable by chemo. He has had multiple recurrences, all treated surgically, so he has had to disappear from home for months at a time. Apparently they never told their son, Billy, that Dad has cancer; when Dad needs surgery, he just disappears in the hospital for a month or two, and they tell the son that it's orthopedic surgery due to a skiing accident Dad had years ago.

Now Billy is 7, and the mother really wants to tell the kid, but the father refuses. In the session, the father kept saying, "Nobody believes that I have cancer because I look so good!" It's true he looked pretty good—since he's never had chemo he still has his hair, etc.—but facts are facts, and he does have cancer. Finally the wife told her husband quietly, "I think you don't want to tell him because you can't admit to yourself that you have cancer. Maybe you figure that if you don't tell Billy, it isn't real. Well, it's real, and he deserves to know, just like I deserved to know when my mom had cancer but I wasn't given the chance." Her husband blinked at her, speechless. When he finally tells Billy, I bet the truth will hit them both pretty hard.

The next person was a man about our age whose wife has terminal pancreatic cancer. I gather the wife goes in and out of consciousness, and he doesn't know what or how to tell their four-year-old daughter. She had drawn a picture for her mother, a crayon drawing of the family, but her mother could not recognize what it was. He brought in the picture to show us, holding it with the tenderness that he obviously feels for his wife and daughter. He looked lost and afraid; he clearly loved his daughter very much, but did not know how to help her.

David and I went last. I said I have lymphoma and about to have brain surgery and start chemo, and we are trying to figure out how to tell our teenage kids. He just said, "I'm David, and I'm Laura's husband." David is a private person, especially with people he doesn't know. I knew that sharing the intimate details of his personal life with strangers at a seminar wasn't his style; he was there for me.

The social worker who ran the meeting was named Tara, which made me think of *Gone with the Wind*. She was young— maybe in her mid thirties—with short dark hair and sparkly eyes. She said she had been working with cancer patients and families for ten years, and that we would tailor the discussion toward the issues confronting the people in the seminar.

After the introductions, Tara gave us a bunch of "How to Tell Your Kids You Have Cancer" literature. Some of it was geared towards very young kids, which won't work for Nate at age 17 and Emma at age 14. For example, they had an interactive workbook with a colorful cover and outlines of a female body, so your kids can draw where Mommy's cancer is; there was also a "his" version with a male body to use if they want to draw Daddy's cancer. We had the oldest kids in the room, and we were the only ones who were there before cancer treatment started—everyone else had been weaving elaborate webs of deception for months or years.

"Be honest, but don't overload the kids with information," Tara explained with a faint southern drawl. "You want to answer their questions, and make it clear that throughout all this, you're still their parents, and you'll take care of them." She emphasized the importance of having time together as a family. In the cab on the way home, David and I talked about how lucky we are to be on the same page about how and what to tell the kids, but we've been on the same page for most of the 31 years we've known each other. We're planning to tell the kids tomorrow. I wish I didn't have to rock their world. But it would rock their world more if I'm not around, and I have to do this chemo to stick around, and I'm going to do whatever it takes.

Wednesday I had pre-admission tests, including an echocardiogram and an EKG to make sure my heart's OK. Thursday I went to the dentist for a pre-chemo cleaning of my teeth. Unfortunately they found two cavities, so I had to have them filled. I'm trying to seal up all potential portals of infection—I feel like I'm drawing up the drawbridges of some ancient castle.

Maureen had told me about the wig store on the West Side that she used when she had chemo, and she met me there Thursday afternoon. When I entered the store, a gay cross-dressing hair stylist named J.T., who has won Emmies for hair design, put me in a little room. I was wearing a green skirt, a sweater, and my Ugg boots. My hair is even longer than the last time you saw me, about five inches below my shoulders, curly brown with more flecks of gray than you remember, and kind of wild. J.T. took one look at me and said, "You're a low maintenance kind of gal, huh?" I laughed and asked, "Isn't it enough that I have cancer and need chemo and now you're dissing my hair?"

I tried on a few brunette wigs, and the two I liked best were long—one curly and one straight. I told J.T. I wanted to try a blonde wig because it was my chance to see if blondes have more fun. He said, "Honey, I've been blonde, and trust me, they DON'T." J.T. has named all the wigs—the curly one was Chelsea, named for Chelsea Clinton, and the straight one was Jennifer (maybe for Jennifer Garner?) and actually looks more like your hair than mine. I gather I'll lose my hair about a month after the chemo starts. Then I go back to the wig place, they cut off the rest of my hair, and I go home wearing one of the wigs.

Yesterday, I went on a "field trip" to see our new suite of offices with our office assistant, Lea. The building has been there awhile, but they just finished construction on our suite, and nobody has moved in yet. I had heard the building was a dump, with no security guard. Apparently there was a report of a flasher in the stairway two weeks ago, and when I told one of the administrators, she said, "Great, now you guys will have entertainment." I've since heard that the woman who saw the flasher "wasn't sure he was flashing." How can you be uncertain about that? It seems to me that if you see a guy in the stairway with his trousers unzipped, there are two options: either he's flashing or he's peeing, and neither is something you want a guy to do in your stairway.

Anyway, the suite was beautiful—lots of light, big central space with offices all around, plenty of computers, a small kitchen area, two bathrooms, and a high-tech conference room. Best of all—the office they have planned for me has real windows! It is so sunny compared to our old suite, and much more spacious. I thought I'd never go there, but now I think I will. It will be a beautiful, quiet place to write.

Today Nate takes his SATs—I hope so much for his sake that they go OK. Tomorrow David and I tell the kids, and Monday I get admitted for the neurosurgery. If all goes well, I come home on Tuesday night, rest Wednesday, and have my first chemo on Thurs 3/15.

Got to go—Nate's up and it's time for the pre-SAT breakfast! Keep writing—I love your letters.

Love
Laura

From: Laura
Sent: Sunday, March 11, 2007 11:29 PM
To: Jennifer
Subject: Telling the kids

Hi Jen. Remember the time a couple of years ago, when you cut back on your office hours to make your child psych practice part-time, four days a week, after Sophie was born? You told me then that you thought you had found the right balance, and I told you how few women ever get to say that. I think it's great that you're thinking of cutting back on work from four to three days a week after the new baby. This balance thing is a moving target. As soon as you get it right, something in life shifts, like a new baby, or aging parents, or moving to a new city, or an illness, and you have to go with it. I read in an article that people are calling it "work-life fit" instead of "work-life balance" these days, because we now recognize that balance is generally unattainable.

We actually told the kids yesterday, rather than today as we had planned. Nate felt good about his SATs, and we were all together. I was in the bedroom with David and I told him that it felt like the right time to tell them, and that letting them know today will give them a little more time to deal with it before the surgery. It would also let them see me go to bed and wake up at home in the morning, a little bit of normal before Armageddon. David agreed.

After dinner we were all sitting in the family room. You wouldn't recognize the kids, Jen—they've gotten so big! Nate is taller than I am, with sandy hair that always looks a little tousled, an athletic build, and those green eyes he got from David. Emma is petite, about 5'2", and incredibly chic; her eyes are still that combination of green and blue, half David's and half mine (all hers). She's wearing her brown hair shorter now, in wisps around her face, and layers her clothes. I love how she wears jewelry—she'll have multiple necklaces, all different, but they look great together, and she prefers wearing a different earring in each ear ("I don't like symmetry," she explains). I sat on the couch, with Nate on my left and Emma on my right, holding both of their hands. David sat in a chair right next to us. I told them that I have lymphoma, a type of cancer, and that it's in my lymph nodes, bone marrow, spinal cord, and the fluid around my brain.

I explained that I need six months of chemotherapy, which is strong medicine to kill the cancer cells. I said that I was going to get chemo at least every two weeks, and for every other one I have to get admitted to the hospital for a few days. I told them that the chemo will make me look sick because I'll lose my hair but that just means the chemo is working. I assured them that cancer is not contagious, that they can't catch it, that they didn't give it to me, that it's nobody's fault, these things just happen. I said that they could talk to anyone they liked about it, that it was no secret, and that I had gotten names for each of them of a psychiatrist they could talk to if they wanted. I told them that we were still their parents, that we would take care of them, and that David is the best dad in the world.

I told them that some people with cancer are cured, some get better, some stay the same, some get sicker, and some die. I told them that my hospital and my doctors were the best on the planet, that I was going to do what the doctors told me, and that I would do everything in my power to be in the group that gets better, and that they know how stubborn I can be! I told them that I needed to have a tube in my chest and one in my head for the chemo, and that I was getting admitted to the hospital on Monday for one night to get the tube in my head. I reminded them that their Aunt Laura survived cancer, and so did their Grandma. And I repeated what I said to my beautiful sister-in-law when she was diagnosed with cancer: it sucks but we'll get through it. She did, and so will we.

David didn't say much during the whole exchange, but he was there, quietly lending support for all of us. His response made me think of our wedding in his parents' house on Long Island. It was time for each of us to have a sip of red wine. Even though we had known each other for six years and lived together for two, I was shaking so hard that I could hardly hold the glass. He reached up and steadied my hands for me, so I could have a drink without spilling wine on my dress or dropping the glass. He has always been there, quietly strong. We're going to need that now more than ever.

Later that night, David and I spoke to each of them separately. Emma wanted details, including a full explanation, complete with diagrams, of where the lymphoma was, where all the tubes were going to be, how many chemos I needed, and what the treatments would involve. Nate just got pale and serious, held my hand, and said, "I love you, Mom."

The kids have always had their own distinct ways of processing information. I remember a day more than a decade ago when we passed a dead bird on the street while we were walking to school. Emma asked questions: "What is that? Is that a dead bird? Why did the bird die?" Nate became silent and asked Emma to please stop talking about it. Emma deals with her fears by verbalizing them and seeking clarification, while Nate prefers to receive information only on a "need to know" basis. After we spoke to the kids, Emma went into Nate's room and they talked in private. David and I thought that was a good sign that the kids will help each other through this.

On Sunday we looked at some college application materials with Nate, and I took Emma out to tea. After we got home, Emma and Nate spent most of the rest of the day downloading iTunes on my computer to put on my iPod. David had the brilliant idea to get me an iPod and have the kids put songs on it so I can listen to music while I'm getting chemo. It's great because when they asked what they could do to help me, we had something to suggest that actually will be helpful. Emma's selections focused on Broadway musicals like Wicked and Spring Awakening, while Nate's had a heavy Motown emphasis, including Marvin Gaye and the Temptations. David put music on for me too—including jazz, which is still his passion, and some classical music that he knows I love.

I called my mom tonight to tell her. She recently moved from the house where I grew up in Newton, Massachusetts to a beautiful retirement community outside of Boston. I didn't want to worry her, but there's no way I can go through this without telling her. She asked me what she can do to help, and I asked her to email me. She said she'll send me a Blue Mountain card every day. I love those e-cards, with their pictures and music.

The brain surgery part is daunting. I've gotten used to my brain the way it is. I'm afraid I won't be me anymore.

Love
Laura

Chapter 3
Treatment Begins

Keep your sense of humor. Discover your inner Zen.
Bring your own anesthesia.

From: Laura
Sent: Monday, March 12, 2007 11:04 PM
To: Jennifer
Subject: Brain surgery

Hi Jen. I survived brain surgery! The neurosurgeon promised he didn't go anywhere near my sense of humor.

Love
Laura

From: Emma
Sent: Tuesday, March 13, 2007 8:14 AM
To: Mom
Subject: For you in the hospital

Guess what!
I love you!
Guess what else!
I couldn't think of anything else.
I love you!

Love
Emma

From: Laura
Sent: Wednesday, March 14, 2007 11:04 PM
To: Jennifer
Subject: Stories

Hi Jen. Here's a story for you. As I was getting ready to go to the OR for the Omaya, they told me I had to take off my underpants. Have you ever seen hospital-issued one-size-fits-none underpants? They are made of such a fine mesh that when you put them on a human body, they are actually clear! The nurse wouldn't give me the clear panties unless I was menstruating, so I looked the nurse in the eye and said I had my period, a lie I haven't told since I wanted to get out of junior high gym. Nothing says "vulnerable" like losing your skivvies. I told the nurse that if the doctor had to look in my underwear to find where to put the Omaya, he wasn't half the neurosurgeon I thought he was. The nurse looked puzzled; I don't think the neurosurgery patients here tell a lot of jokes.

The surgery part was bizarre. Completely awake, I walked down the hall with the escort guy when it was time for my brain surgery. I had to remove my glasses—more vulnerability, especially if you're almost legally blind without them. David walked with us at first, but when we got to the door of the operating room area, he had to turn back. I went into the OR, which was full of shiny instruments, harsh overhead lights, and "the wall of knowledge"—a huge computer screen to provide continuous updates of the patient's pulse, temperature, blood pressure, oxygenation, and other parameters—and I realized that soon it would be my information up there. I had to climb onto the table and lie down. The anesthesiologist gave me good drugs that put me to sleep. The next thing I remember is waking up in my room after the surgery was done, with a bad headache and an even worse hair day—they'd shaved almost a quarter of my hair.

Did you know that an iPod is a great cancer coping strategy? I have 370 songs on it, courtesy of Emma, Nate, and David. Waiting for and recovering from brain surgery are a whole lot less scary when you've got headphones in and you're listening to Ben E. King singing "Stand By Me."

Love
Laura

From: Laura
Sent: Thursday, March 15, 2007 10:43 PM
To: Jennifer
Subject: Where's the Zen?

Hi Jen—You are my most faithful correspondent!

After my first inpatient experience, what I want to know is, how am I going to find the Zen to get through this treatment? When I was first diagnosed, David and I decided that we needed to look deep inside ourselves and find some inner Zen and patience, because being a patient involves a lot of waiting. If I fight everything every step of the way, it will zap all of my energy and I won't have any left to use to fight the lymphoma.

And yet in the hospital, when I had to explain to a nurse who looked 12 years old at 3 am how to diagnose an infiltrated IV ("See, the left arm is now twice as big as the right, and my watch is making a huge dent in my arm, and you can see the indentation in my left ring finger, which looks like a sausage now, from where my wedding rings used to be before I took them off so you wouldn't have to cut them off in the morning"), or wait an additional three hours after the neurosurgeon told me I could go home while somebody fills out pointless paperwork, I couldn't hold onto the Zen even for 24 hours. But I need to find that Zen. I can't waste energy on stupid stuff, because I need to save it for what counts. A patient told me that every time I go to the hospital I should pretend I'm going to the airport, so I expect a long wait. That way, I'll be pleasantly surprised if I don't wait rather than disappointed if I do. I'll try it.

After the IV infiltrated during my admission, they were going to stick me again because I needed one more dose of IV antibiotics, and I asked the 12-year-old nurse if she could please just use the Mediport in my chest. She said she wasn't sure, and would have to check with the nursing supervisor. I told her that the Interventional Radiology (IR) doc who put in the port said they could use it during this admission and so did the neurosurgeon, but she insisted that she could only do it if the nursing supervisor blessed it. I emailed the IR docs, my neurosurgeon, and my lymphoma doc to ask if they would bless using the port, and if so, could they let the nurses on 7 know? Miracle of miracles, the nurse came back and said they could use the port!

Innocently, I had always thought that once a port is in, that getting injected through the port would feel the same as injecting IV tubing after the IV is already in place—ie, painless. Unfortunately, the port is under a tiny layer of skin which has lots of nerve endings. The term "access the port" is a euphemism for "I'm going to take a dagger and stab you in the heart." No local anesthesia of any kind—no injection, no cream, no freezing spray, nothing. It made me appreciate how much pain patients go through with the procedures we inflict on them. And then the nurse bragged about how she was the best in her nursing school class at accessing the port! For every patient to whom I ever said that the injection of anesthetic was more painful than the needle stick for the procedure, I am paying my penance to the universe.

And yet, during the same admission, I experienced a precious act of kindness. The morning after the Omaya placement, a nurses' aide asked if I'd like her help washing up, and I gratefully said yes. I got undressed and sat on a little plastic chair. She gently and respectfully assisted me with the hand-held nozzle that controlled the wonderful flow of hot water while keeping my post-op head dry. It's pretty intimate and potentially awkward to bathe in front of a stranger, but she made it so simple. This woman, a non-native speaker of the English language without much formal education, was everything you could want in a caregiver. I wish I could triple her salary.

Today, at home, the part of my hair that wasn't shaved was all tangled in knots that I didn't see how I could fix, especially since I can't take a real shower for a few days because of the neurosurgery. Carmen, our wonderful nanny from Jamaica who has been taking care of the kids for thirteen years, was there. I told you the story about how we got Carmen, didn't I? We found Carmen through friends who had hired her temporarily when their nanny was on vacation; she was their nanny's cousin. When we interviewed Carmen, I felt an instant connection. We hired her on the spot, and she's been with us since Emma was 18 months old and Nate was three. She's part of our family—great with the kids. I love to talk to her when I get home and have her tell me stories about what the kids did during the day.

When I got home from the neurosurgery admission, Carmen and I were the only ones there; the kids were still at school. I asked Carmen to help me cut off some of the tangled hair before the kids got home. We went into the bedroom and she cut a few snips. Clumps of hair fell like parts of a bird's nest on the bed. Afterwards, I saw that even a "combover" doesn't cover the shaved part of my head, which looks like Frankenstein: at the site of the Omaya, I have staples, bruising, and a big bump. It's a little scary even for me; the kids would not like it. As Carmen was finishing up, we heard the front door slam; Nate was home. I quickly searched my closet, put on a Yankee's cap, and went to kiss him hello while Carmen threw away the evidence. I suppose eventually the kids will have to see my head, but not now, not yet.

Today, I was scheduled to get my first intrathecal chemo injected into the Omaya and then my first IV R-CHOP. After experiencing the pain from having the Mediport accessed, I decided I would bring my own anesthesia. I brought a bottle of Gebauer's Ethyl Chloride spray, a freezing spray that numbs instantly. As a doctor, I had been using Ethyl Chloride spray for years to numb the breast during pre-operative needle localizations, a procedure in which we put a wire in the breast to guide a surgeon to a breast abnormality that can't be felt. I also brought a tube of Emla cream, another medication that numbs the skin but takes half an hour to work.

When I went to the lymphoma service and they described how they were going to stick the Omaya, I asked if they used anesthesia. To give an intrathecal injection, they need to put a needle into the Omaya; since the part they inject is sewn under your scalp, you can feel it. They told me that this area "cannot be numbed." I pulled out the bottle of Ethyl Chloride spray and said, "Actually, it can!" I explained that we use this spray in Mammo for needle locs and that it really helps ease the pain. I asked if they could please use it for me, and they did. After the spray, my oncologist and another very experienced doc dug around my head with a needle for about 10-15 minutes and couldn't find the Omaya, so they gave up. If I hadn't had the spray, it would have been torture.

I have to go back Tuesday for them to try again; I've invited the neurosurgeon to join us, so he can show them where to go (I'd like to tell them where to go!), and he has agreed to come. I think part of the problem is that the neurosurgeons put the Omayas in but the oncologists inject them. Since neurosurgery only puts in about 20 Omayas a year, and there are far more than 20 oncologists, most oncologists don't have much experience with intrathecal injections. When the oncologist recommended that I bring the spray on Tuesday (which I will do—I'm bringing it everywhere from now on), I suggested that maybe it would be good to get some spray for the clinic, so that all patients would benefit! Patients rarely come armed with their own anesthetic spray. I hope you never get cancer, but if you ever do, don't leave home without the spray.

I had a blood test and then went to the outpatient chemo floor to get my first R-CHOP. Waiting for chemo felt like being in line for a table at a crowded restaurant—they asked for my cell number, so they could call me when the chemo was ready. They wait for the blood test results before they "mix the chemo," which then takes an additional two hours after the blood test result is ready. They want to make sure that your blood counts are normal before they give you chemo. While I was waiting, I got to have breakfast with David. Finally, they called around 12:30, and we got started.

I went up to the 4th floor, Suite 7. It's outpatient chemo, but it looks like an inpatient floor. The room was private, with a bed, two chairs, a TV, and a private bathroom. I had brought a fuzzy turquoise blanket from home. My nurse was named Lois,

31

and she was very nice. She used the spray on my port before she "accessed it" and she laughed at my jokes even though I doubt that they were funny. They run in the first chemo slowly, over 6-8 hours, so they can monitor for an allergic reaction. They started with the Benadryl (anti-histamine), Dexamethasone (an injectable steroid), and a slew of anti-nausea pre-meds in preparation for the Rituximab (monoclonal antibody), followed by the cytoxan with a lot of fluid, the doxorubicin (which is bright red and will make me pee pink!), and the vincristine.

The problem with most chemo is that it works by killing rapidly dividing cells. Cancer cells divide rapidly, so chemo can kill cancer, but unfortunately some normal cells also divide rapidly, like the cells that make hair, causing hair loss; and the cells that become blood cells, including red blood cells, so you get anemic; platelets, so you have a tendency to bleed; and white blood cells, so you're prone to infection. Giving chemo is the ultimate game of chicken—you explode a big bomb in the patient and wait to see who dies first, the cancer or the patient.

The complications of chemo that can kill you are mostly related to the innocent bystanders like white blood cells who get hit in the cross-fire. Now there are medicines that are "growth factors" that help some "good cells," like blood cells, recover faster, so a cancer patient is vulnerable for a shorter period of time; this has greatly helped survival. Hopefully in the future we'll have more "targeted therapies"—medicines that will specifically attack the cancer cells, while leaving the innocent bystanders alone. Unfortunately, now we usually still explode the bomb.

David stayed with me the whole day. He was in a chair, reading. He loves to read Big Fat Books—I call them BFBs—it started with that multi-volume biography of Lyndon Johnson by Robert Caro a few years back and has continued since then—I worry that he will fall asleep with one of those humungous tomes and will suffer a BFB injury! Some friends from the hospital came to see me, including Cindy, our Chief Technologist in Breast Imaging, whom I've known since we both started working at Memorial 17 years ago.

Nate visited me after school. He was on his way to Pediatrics in my hospital to interview for a volunteer position dealing with children who have cancer. Working in Peds was Nate's idea—he loves to work with children. I think it's a great idea for that reason and also because it might help him cope with my illness. He likes to deal with a difficult experience by turning it into a way he can help other people. I hope it won't be too tough on him emotionally; some of those kids with cancer are really sick.

I did fine with the chemo—no reactions or anything— and was done earlier than expected, 6:30 instead of 8:30 pm. So now we're home, and I can rest. If I feel up to it I may go to the office tomorrow. Apparently I won't get to "nadir," which is the lowest point in the white blood cell count, for about a week; that's when I'll be particularly susceptible to infection. They say that the effect of chemo is cumulative; it's likely that I'll feel more exhausted after more chemos. The doctors think I'll need a total of 18 treatments (six outpatient IV R-CHOPS for the nodes and marrow, six outpatient intrathecal methotrexates for the fluid around my brain, and six inpatient IV methotrexates for the spinal cord disease), so now I just have 17 left.

Keep writing. It makes sense that you're not accepting new patients for now—that will make it easier for you to make the switch from four to three days a week when the time comes. And I agree that having it all may not be what it's cracked up to be. As the great comedian Steven Wright says, "You can't have everything—where would you put it?"

Love
Laura

From: Laura
Sent: Friday, March 16, 2007 8:56 AM
To: Jennifer
Subject: Home

Today I'm home resting. Emma has a snow day so she's home too. We're listening to the CD of a Broadway musical we're seeing next month called Spring Awakening. We're going to make some tea and have a cozy day together.

Love
Laura

From: Laura
Sent: Saturday, March 17, 2007 4:14 AM
To: Jennifer
Subject: Awake

Hi Jen. I have a feeling there may be quite a few 3-5 am updates, especially when I'm on prednisone, the oral steroid I have to take for about five days after every R-CHOP (I hear prednisone is a good medicine to take when you need to clean your apartment). The prednisone seems to wake me up from 3:00 to 5:00 am even though I'm on enough sleep meds to kill a pretty large race horse. I guess it will help me get a jump start on my book.

I'm going to listen to music and try to get back to sleep. I'm in the mood to hear Jacqueline du Pre play her rich and passionate performance of Elgar's cello concerto. I remember the stories you told me about Jacqueline du Pre: how she used to play duets with her husband, Daniel Barenboim, who was a pianist and conductor; how she developed multiple sclerosis, making her unable to play the cello; and how the rest of her life after that was very rough. Knowing about her illness, I found it sad to read the back cover of the CD, which reports an interview her husband gave before she got sick, when he said that the best thing about their relationship was that "our life and work are one."

Love
Laura

From: Laura
Sent: Saturday, March 17, 2007 11:20 AM
To: Radiology staff
Subject: Thank you

Dear Radiology colleagues:
      Thank you for the beautiful gift basket, and the note that accompanied it. As many of you know, I have an aggressive lymphoma and need six months of intensive chemo. If all goes well, I'll be done with the chemo by September.
      After four years as an intern/resident at MSKCC and 17 years on faculty here, I finally get to see what it's like to be a cancer patient. You know that song, "I'd rather be a hammer than a nail"? Well, yes I would! Anyway, I'm writing a book about it. You know I love to write.

I appreciate your kind wishes and (if you're up for it) your prayers. My wonderful family and friends are helping me get through this. Thank you.

Love
Laura

From: Laura
Sent: Sunday, March 18, 2007 9:07 AM
To: Jennifer
Subject: Shower

Hi Jen. Guess what? Yesterday I got to take my first real shower since I had neurosurgery! My being unable to shower for five days was a true test of my husband's love, and I'm delighted that he passed.

The neurosurgeon told me to use Baby Shampoo, so David went out to get it for me. He came back with a bottle of Johnson's baby shampoo with a Spanish label that said something about "mata" on the front. In Spanish, matar means to kill, so I told my husband, I send you out and you come back with death shampoo? I told the kids if they heard any explosions from the bathroom they should come in with a hose. So my poor darling husband went out again (I was really just kidding) and came back with two bottles of Johnson's Baby Shampoo, both labeled in English (one had a Detangling Formula). Neither mentioned death in any language anywhere on the label. I was surprised they had Baby Detangling Shampoo; I never thought babies got tangles—maybe they don't, which is why there were so many bottles left in the store!

What a shower it was. Feeling the warm water cascading over my head, I closed my eyes and recalled the first time I went snorkeling in the balmy turquoise waters of the Caribbean.

Tonight we're going out for a surprise party for my husband's 50th birthday. The last time I tried to give him a surprise birthday party was when we were in college. I had bought him a cake and lit the candles in the dorm room of his friend, an Egyptian named Sammy. Trying to convince David to come to his room, Sammy said, "David, I have to talk to you in my room!" and David asked, "Why not tell me here?" and refused to come until Sammy spilled the beans! The candles were all burned down into wax on the cake by the time they showed up. I had sworn never again. But that was about 30 years ago, and I figured that the statute of limitations should have expired by now.

Love
Laura

Chapter 4
Celebration

It's not all about the cancer.

From: Laura
Sent: Monday, March 19, 2007 4:36 AM
To: Jennifer
Subject: David's birthday party

Hi Jen. Since you're my "gentle reader," let me tell you about David's 50th birthday party last night. (Note the ungodly time on the email; I'm still on the five days of prednisone from the R-CHOP, and it continues to get me up from 3-5 am daily. Maybe I should call my book "The Prednisone Diaries.")

I'd been thinking about throwing a surprise 50th birthday party for David for a long time. A few years ago, we went to a party for our closest friends, the Berkowitzes. Our dear friend Steve Berkowitz turned 50, and his wife Monique (we call her "Q"), threw him a fabulous dinner party that occupied a small floor of a little bistro downtown. Q had invited friends from all times in Steve's life: growing up in Boston, playing in a band, and rising through the record industry in NY. Each of them got up and told moving and funny stories about Steve from his childhood through his adult life. The party inspired me to do something for David's 50th birthday.

I enlisted Q to help me plan the party. Given everything that was going on, we decided to keep it simple, with just the four of us (me, David, Nate, and Emma) and the four of them (Q, Steve, and their sons, Nick and Ben). Our families have been close for years. Our nanny had befriended their nanny in

Carl Schurz Park when Nick and Nate were babies, and the boys bonded right away. I first met Nick when I was pushing Nate, then 18 months old, in his stroller in the park. Nick waved and said, "Hi, Nate!" It was the first time, to my knowledge, that somebody with whom I was unacquainted knew Nate. In that moment, Nick taught me that Nate was someday going to have a full and independent life that did not always include me! Shortly after that, we all met in the park. Q and I became pregnant with our second children at around the same time and became close friends. The eight of us have spent every New Year's Day together for about 15 years, at our place or theirs.

David still loves jazz, and loves to take the kids to jazz clubs. One of his favorite clubs in the city is a funky place called the Jazz Standard, which has great live music and serves dinner. Q and I looked at the schedule of who is playing, and it turns out that this weekend they had a quartet with a pianist named Bill Charlap, who I knew David liked. We decided to do it on Sunday night.

The kids liked the plan, especially the part about keeping it a surprise from David. Nate tried to help me make the reservations, but when he told them it was for a party of eight, they said you can't make reservations for 8 people. So I called back the manager and said, "Listen, I have cancer, and we need to celebrate my husband's 50th birthday on Sunday because after that I'll be hospitalized." And guess what? It turns out that you CAN make reservations for eight people! So cancer is a good news/bad news thing. Yes, you need toxic chemo—but at least now you can get dinner reservations!

I booked us for the 7:30 set and finalized the plans for Steve, Q, and their kids to meet us there. I had casually mentioned to David earlier in the week that maybe we could go out to eat on Sunday for brunch or dinner. He said dinner is better because the kids need to do their homework during the day (I had been counting on him saying that). Emma overheard the conversation. After David left the room, Emma looked at me admiringly. "Mom, if I had a hat, I would take it off to you."

When Sunday came, David was full speed ahead in superdrive mode to make sure that the kids got their homework done, and he said he wasn't sure we'd have time to go out to dinner. Emma was worried—what if we can't talk Dad into going? But I reassured Emma by reminding her of the line in My Big Fat Greek Wedding where the Greek mom says that the man of the house may be the head, but the woman is the neck, and she can turn the head whichever way she wants.

Here's how it went down. About 5:45 I was alone in the family room and David came in and asked, "Where are we going for dinner?" When I hedged, he began to suggest restaurants, and then he realized I had a plan. His face was apprehensive and his arms were crossed, something he does in the rare moments when he gets upset. He said he wanted me to tell him what's going on, because he can't deal with any more surprises after the shock of my diagnosis. I told him that I'd made a surprise celebration for his 50th birthday, that we had reservations at the Jazz Standard, that Bill Charlap was playing, that the Berkowitzes were going to meet us there, and that there would be cake and presents. David looked puzzled, like he didn't understand. He asked, "How can I celebrate my birthday and be happy in the middle of all of this?"

I explained it to him. I told him how much fun it had been for all of us to plan this wonderful dinner, how the kids had been bumping into each other for two days trying to keep it a secret. I told him that we can't make the next six months of our lives all about the cancer. That one of the things that will get us through this is to find the moments in our lives that deserve to be celebrated and to celebrate them. That he was having a birthday, and that Emma is going to Paris for her spring break, that Nate survived the SATs, that I finished 1 of my 18 chemos (only 17 left!), and that after 24 years of marriage we're still together.

We got in the cab, and Nate gave the driver the address. The Berkowitzes met us in the narrow entryway of the jazz club and I said: "Recipe for instant party: add four Berkowitzes, and let the fun begin!" The eight of us went downstairs to the dimly lit foyer. The restaurant had a sprinkling of small tables and booths with an elevated stage in the front, and the walls were covered with signed photographs of jazz giants who had played there in the past. They seated us at a table with a long curvy booth on the left and cushioned chairs on the right, so we could all be comfortable. David and I were in the middle of the table, between the senior Berkowitzes and all the kids.

One of the most wonderful things about the party was how we're all so close—some of us got up and moved around to different seats, so by the end of the evening, everybody had talked to everybody. It's so rare in relationships among eight people that all of the possible combinations work, but with our two families, they always have. Good food, great music, and then they brought out the chocolate cake that said "Happy 50th Birthday David" that we had pre-ordered with one candle. I decided not to put in 50 candles, remembering the debacle of the waxed cake from David's college days.

I couldn't resist making a little speech. David is always teasing me about how I tell the long version of the story, never the short version. He likes to tell me the Colin Quinn joke about his girlfriend telling him an interminable story with every possible detail included, and Colin says to her, "Excuse me, but I don't want to live your life in real time!" I kept my remarks short and sweet. I thanked everyone for coming and said how glad I was that we could all be here for David's birthday. Then we drank a toast to wish David a happy birthday—the boys did it with Coke, and Emma had a sip of champagne.

At home, after the kids went to bed, David thanked me and said it was "good to have the distraction for the kids." But it's more than that. We live our lives too fast, and don't look around enough. I realized it once when I was dashing through the reef while scuba diving, as if I had to make some deadline. You're in the water and the coral reef is magnificent; you might as well enjoy the view. The good things are not a distraction. They're the point. David has been saying that for years, and I believed him in theory, but didn't really live my life that way. I'm finally getting it. It's ironic that I'm teaching David the lesson he's been trying to teach me for three decades.

On another note—I can't believe you and Sophie watched The Devil Wears Prada last night—Emma & I were watching it too! We just got the DVD. We had seen the movie in the theater in Hilton Head this summer—but the problem with seeing it in Hilton Head is that it instills in you the longing to shop in New York, which is tough to do when you're in South Carolina.

Tomorrow I'm going to work, and then Tuesday intrathecal methotrexate. If they can't find the Omaya this time I'm going over to the mammo office so Cindy can do an ultrasound and draw a big arrow on my head.

Love
Laura

From: Laura
Sent: Tuesday, March 20, 2007 5:29 AM

42

To: Jennifer
Subject: The Prednisone Diaries

Hi Jen. This may be the last installment of "The
Prednisone Diaries" (3-5 am version) for awhile. Today will be
my last day of oral prednisone for this cycle. I take it for the
first 5 days after the R-CHOP, and today will be day 5. And
darn, I had hoped I'd get the whole apartment cleaned while on
that steroid rush! Imagine how clean Mark Maguire's apartment
must be.

Yesterday was the first day I really went back to work
since the surgery. It was a Monday, and on Mondays and
Wednesdays I direct the Program for Women Faculty Affairs.
I'd love to show you my office. After you go in the front door,
there is a kitchen to the immediate right, and past the kitchen is
the door to our suite. My office has a desk, bookcases, a round
table that can fit three chairs easily, and a window overlooking
some trees on the street, my first office window in over 17
years.

I had a bunch of stuff to do in the office, but I took it
slow. I had to finalize some details for this Wednesday's
breakfast meeting of Athena, which is our informal group for
women faculty. We call this group Athena after the Greek
goddess of wisdom and war. In Homer's Odyssey, Odysseus
asks a wise and trusted old man named Mentor to take care of
his son Telemachus when Odysseus goes off to fight the Trojan
War. It turns out it is actually Athena, a woman and a goddess,
disguised as Mentor, who guides Telemachus in the Odyssey.
We thought Athena was the perfect name for a group of women
faculty who offer each other support and guidance.

Cindy came to see me in the Women's Office. She
brought me a maroon baseball cap that said "Monk," after the
detective with obsessive compulsive disorder (OCD) who is the

hero of my favorite TV show. Monk's OCD makes him a great detective, because he notices everything, but complicates his life because of his many phobias and rituals. Cindy is a cancer survivor, and last year, when she was recovering after surgery, I sent her a collection of Monk DVDs. It seems right that now that I have cancer, she gave me a Monk cap. A few other friends had sent gifts to the office. One of the good things about having cancer is that people are always giving you "cancer presents." It's like Christmas in the spring!

I figured out a plan to structure my days for the immediate future. On Mondays and Wednesdays if I'm up to it, I'll go to the Women's Office. The other days, if I'm not getting treated or hospitalized, I'll go to my Radiology office to do some administrative work or research. I'll aim to leave work at 4 pm, so I can be here when the kids get home from school. Jen, I'm almost 47, my kids are 17 and 14, and yesterday, when they came home from 11th and 9th grade respectively, I got to offer them milk and cookies and ask them about their day at school. Finally!

When I got home yesterday, I talked to Carmen. I asked her how she thought the kids were doing through all of this. She said that it's hard on them but they'll be OK. She told me how much time the kids spend with each other at home these days, talking in Nate's room with the door closed. I was relieved to hear it. How wonderful if they can support each other. Around 4:30, the kids came home; Emma settled down to schoolwork and Nate closed the door in his room to take a nap.

I went to the laptop to write; Carmen gave me a hug and left. The laptop is on the dining table in our living room, which we redecorated since you last saw it. It still has bookcases on most of the walls, the dining table on the near right, and the piano on the left. We got shades to cover most of the glass windows on the far side of the living room, but left bare the glass door that opens onto the terrace. We bought a big Oriental rug. We also replaced the old couch with an oversized sofa that has big stuffed pillows and got two comfy "glider" chairs in muted colors with a hint of turquoise. I love to sit in one of the gliders and read and listen to David playing the piano. Around 6 pm, the kids emerged from their rooms, hungry for dinner.

We ordered dinner from a neighborhood Italian place called Arturo's, one of our family favorites. I called David on his cell to ask what he wanted me to order for him, and he was glad that I was home. We had a family dinner for a change, and then the kids escaped to their homework. That little extra time with the kids when they get home from school and having dinner all together felt like a gift—I usually don't get home until after seven. Later I told David that for the next few months I would try to get home before the kids whenever possible, and he said that sounded like a good idea.

Today they're going to make a second attempt to give me intrathecal methotrexate in the Omaya. David asked me what time the appointment was so he could reschedule his day to come with me, but I don't want to drag him to all my appointments. He has to work, take care of the kids, and handle the logistics of our lives. If I really need him, like I did when I had brain surgery, I won't hesitate to ask, but if it's not essential, I'd rather conserve his energy. Cindy offered to come with me and sounded like she meant it, so I think I'll take her up on it.

The prednisone buzz is fading, and I may go back to sleep for a little while.

More tomorrow.

Love
Laura

From: Laura
Sent: Tuesday, March 20, 2007 11:14 PM
To: Cindy
Subject: Oh Me Omaya

Hi Cinderella. Just a note to thank you for your starring role in the drama "Oh Me Omaya." I appreciate your coming with me for the intrathecal injection today. You were exactly the right person to be there for me when I needed you, and I will never forget it.

Love
Laura

From: Laura
Sent: Wednesday, March 21, 2007 6:26 AM
To: Jennifer
Subject: Intrathecal chemo: it worked!

Hi J. Yesterday I went to the hospital for intrathecal chemo. The neurosurgeon made his guest appearance and showed the oncologist where to go. Cindy came with me. I figured since she's expert at using the numbing spray from having participated in thousands of breast localizations, she could jump up and spray my head if necessary.

I instinctively reached out to Cindy, and she was a good choice. We started at Memorial around the same time 17 years ago, when I was a fledgling radiologist and she was a breast imaging technologist who worked with our mobile van mammography screening program. Since that time, she has risen through the ranks and is now the Chief Technologist of Breast Imaging at Memorial Hospital. You haven't met her— she has blonde hair and looks like Cameron Diaz. In fact, before she became a radiology technologist, she used to be a hand model!

Cindy and I seem to be there for each other at key moments in our lives. Two years ago I came to the office on a vacation day morning to tidy up some loose ends. I called Cindy in the mammography office about some work-related issue, and she told me she had a new breast lump. I read her mammogram, did a breast ultrasound and a needle biopsy that day, and referred her to the breast surgeon who cured her breast cancer. And now Cindy's there for me.

When I introduced her to my oncologist, I said "This is Cindy, the Chief Technologist in Breast Imaging" and he asked her, "Can you help me schedule a mammogram on one of my patients?" Without missing a beat, Cindy said, "Sure, but only if you get this tap on the first try!" Go Cindy! I could have kissed her feet. They got it and gave me the chemo. I felt nauseated afterwards and had to lie down. Cindy was great—she stayed with me and held my hand while I was getting the chemo and took me home in a cab. When we were in my building, Cindy took me upstairs; I introduced her to Nate, Emma, and Carmen, and then I went to lie down.

Now I have to go, because we're having an Athena breakfast 7-9 am today to celebrate recent women's appointments and promotions. If I feel up to it, I'll stay at work for awhile afterwards; otherwise, I'll come home, and go back to sleep. Phil, the oncologist, wants to give me intrathecal twice a week (Tues/Thurs) for the next 3-4 weeks, until the CSF "clears" (which means has no more malignant cells), and then we'll see.

Love
Laura

From: Laura
Sent: Thursday, March 22, 2007 2:16 AM
To: Jennifer
Subject: Athena breakfast

Hi Jen. The Athena breakfast yesterday was OK. We have these Athena events once a month. We usually meet from 5-7 pm, but sometimes we have an early breakfast or lunch, so that women with different schedules can come. Athena is a chance for women faculty and administrators from MSKCC to meet informally. Before each Athena, I get a list of all the recent women faculty appointments and promotions (A&Ps), and then I invite those women to Athena to celebrate. We get RSVPs so we know who's coming, and we have a little celebration in which we give each of them a flower. The event is pretty low-key—people filter in and out as they can.

For the breakfasts, we order food for the number of people coming and it's served buffet style. I usually get there around 7 and put in the CD with the background music. We mill around and eat and chat until 8, and then I take 10-15 minutes to make announcements. I was supposed to be there at 7 today, and actually was up before 6. I had showered to go, but then I felt sick, all sweaty and nauseated and faint, and I had to lie back down. David was surprised—"Weren't you going to get up?" he asked. When I told him I didn't feel well, he helped me crawl back into bed. I asked him to wake me up so I could be at work by 7:45.

When he woke me up at 7 am, I felt better. I showered again and put on nice clothes—a flowing skirt with rust and green flowers, a green shirt, a little green jacket, and my favorite green hat (from Banana Republic). I haven't started losing my hair from the chemo yet, but my head still looks pretty scary, so I'd rather keep it covered. I took a cab to the Boardroom.

When I arrived, about 20 women were there already, and the breakfast buffet was out. Usually we get a continental breakfast, fruit and bagels and pastries, but today we decided on real food—scrambled eggs and home fries. When I entered, people seemed glad to see me. I told them I had brought the background music, and offered them a choice of Murray Perahia playing Mozart Piano Concertos or the Beach Boys Greatest Hits. And guess what? We went with the Beach Boys! That was my first choice too—the Beach Boys got me through the first round of chemo.

After "California Girls," I got up to make the announcements. Usually I stand at the podium, but when I stood up I got lightheaded and dizzy, like I do when I'm dehydrated after spending too much time on the beach in the hot sun, so I sat down. The other women sat in circles at adjacent tables. I made the announcements, which, in another deviation from the norm, I had written out in advance.

"It has become our tradition at Athena to celebrate women faculty achievements at MSKCC, particularly appointments and promotions," I said. "We are blessed to work at the greatest cancer hospital in the world. We save lives, and take away fear, and discover cures, and make the world a better place. And these activities keep us busy, and impact on the rest of our lives. It is important in the midst of all of this work to take a moment to celebrate our achievements and congratulate each other on our successes.

This seems particularly important to me now. As many of you know, I was recently diagnosed with lymphoma and am being treated here at Memorial. I need six months of chemotherapy, and have already finished two treatments. This experience makes me believe even more strongly that we need to savor special moments in our lives as they come. So today we continue our tradition by welcoming women newly appointed and congratulating women recently promoted at Memorial. Please join me in the following celebrations..."

We celebrated each woman's new appointment or promotion by giving her a flower. We passed around a hand-held mike, so that each woman being honored had the chance to speak. I was touched when a terrific surgeon thanked me for my help with her promotion package and my work with women faculty. Then we went back to milling around. I got faint and a nice pediatrician named Yasmin took me home in a cab.

I lay down most of the morning, and must have napped off and on. When I woke up, Carmen was there. I guess she's my nanny now. She was so sweet—she got me water and made me herbal tea. After that I fell asleep for real. By the time I woke up, it was dark outside, and the kids had come home.

Emma had decided to help find me the Zen. She went to Barnes & Noble after school and bought me my own Itty Bitty Buddha, a tiny reddish portly gentleman with gynecomastia (male breasts) and a protuberant belly which apparently brings you luck when you rub it, so rub away I did. Carmen made us dinner, David came home, and Carmen left. I hung out with David and the kids between naps. Emma and I watched the latest installation of America's Next Top Model, and we agreed that we both hate Renee, although she did take a good picture of being dead.

This afternoon I have to get another dose of intrathecal chemo. Cindy will come with me again.

Love
Laura

From: Laura
Sent: Friday, March 23, 2007 6:19 AM
To: Jennifer
Subject: More intrathecal chemo

Dearest Jen,

Notice, first of all, the luxuriously late time on this email—it's after 6 am now! It's hard for me to think that only a few months ago, I would have thought 6 am was early. I woke up at 2 am as usual but had some herb tea and a piece of banana bread that Q had bought for me and went back to sleep, listening to the Brahms Clarinet Trio that you and I used to play with Susan, the clarinetist, before she moved to New Jersey. I woke up again at 5 am, showered, took my pharmacy of morning meds, made more tea, had a piece of fruit (not bad nutrition considering the chemo, right?), and now I'm here writing to you.

Yesterday was a busy day—two appointments, neurosurgery staple removal at 11 am and intrathecal methotrexate at 3 pm. I had been a little worried about the staple removal—I figured it would hurt. I wanted Cindy to come with me for the intrathecal chemo, and I didn't want to ask her to come to both. I asked Q to come to the neurosurgery appointment, although I was afraid it might be too graphic for someone who doesn't work in the hospital, and I figured I'd probably kick her out when the neurosurgeon came in. But it was actually fine—removing the staples took about a minute and didn't hurt at all—it was like taking out a barrette! My

51

neurosurgeon is terrific. I asked how a nice Jewish boy from Tennessee like him got interested in brain surgery, and he replied, "Well, I couldn't sing."

After the staples were out, Q took me home in a cab and came upstairs. Carmen was here by then and had cleaned the place and opened the windows and terrace door, so there was fresh air in the apartment. I lay down on the couch and rested while Q and Carmen made lunch. Q had bought me delicious chicken soup and a soft roll from the Vinegar Factory, which was perfect. And then Q left.

I called my older brother; I'd been meaning to call him for days. He seemed apprehensive until I said to him, "So now I've had brain surgery and they're putting chemo into my brain, and I'm still smarter than you!" He laughed, relieved. If I could still talk trash, I must be OK. I asked him to look after our mom, who lives near him in Massachusetts. We had a nice but brief chat until Emma came home. I talked to Emma for a few minutes about her day in school, and then it was time to for intrathecal chemo.

I met Cindy there around 3. They checked my blood counts with a quick "fingerstick," meaning they just prick your fingertip with a needle. After the results came back, I went in for more intrathecal chemo. The procedure went fine, but afterwards I felt nauseated and I vomited. Wonderful Cindy held my hair back so I wouldn't puke all over it. And another thing I've noticed (as long as I'm using my experience as a patient to revolutionize patient care): have you ever wondered why those tiny little barf basins are so small? Because when you're throwing up, what you really want is not just to puke, but to have to hit a very precise tiny little peanut-shaped target. I asked the nurse, since we're the finest cancer hospital in the world, don't you think that maybe we could spring for the larger basins? Am I the first puking person to ever want a wider net?

I sat with Cindy for a long time. She is brushing up on her "Reiki" which is a kind of massage that is supposed to have a healing touch, and it helps, or she does, or both, I don't know which. Then we went downstairs. I sat in the lobby (68th between 1st & York) while Cindy got a cab.

A physician colleague named Cheryl walked by. I was still nauseated, and had my head between my knees, trying not to throw up again. Cheryl asked how I was, and I told her I had just had chemo and thrown up, and she said, "Have you talked to other patients who have had similar experiences?" I replied that in the 17 years I've been working here, I have talked to a few cancer patients. And she said, "No, I mean now, as a patient? Maybe you should join a support group." I'm sorry, I know she means well, but here's some advice to people who want to help: if your friend with cancer is about to puke, don't refer her to a support group. Just give her a bucket.

Cindy got me a cab (just in the nick of time—I was going to use my last reserve of energy to strangle Cheryl), and she slid in and I climbed after her. When I got home, Nate and Carmen were there and then Emma came. I lay down on the living room couch with the TV on. Nate covered me up with a fuzzy green blanket and I fell asleep.

So the intrathecal methotrexate is a bitch. They want me to take nausea meds before my next treatment on Wednesday. On Thursday I get admitted for the IV methotrexate, which is supposed to be the hardest of all. Phil says I'll be in the hospital at least five days. My spirit can take it but I hope my body's up for it. Bring it on.

Love
Laura

Chapter 5
Hats and Silver Linings

Look at this as an opportunity to get new hats.

From: Laura
Sent: Friday, March 23, 2007 2:03 PM
To: Jennifer
Subject: Hats

Dearest Jen,

Where do I begin to tell the story about the hats? (Love Story music in background.)

Maybe I should start with the diagnosis of cancer, when I realized that I should look upon this not as losing my hair but as an opportunity to buy new hats. And then maybe I'll skip to the point where Emma & I went on-line to look up hats, and found the most beautiful hats I'd ever seen, made by a woman named Christine A. Moore. When I looked up her website, I found she has a studio in New York. She answered my phone call herself. "Christine?" I asked. "Yes?" she replied. "My name is Laura," I explained. "I'd like to come and see your beautiful hats." She said, "Are you a buyer for a store?" I told her that I'm a doctor in a cancer hospital who just became a cancer patient, and if I wear her hats and look fabulous, she will sell a lot of hats. She inquired, "What time would you like to come in?" We arranged it for today at 10 am. Just in time. My 47th birthday is tomorrow, the day my beautiful Emma is going on a class trip to Paris.

Yesterday I called Christine to confirm. Her address was near Macy's on the West Side. Although I had a tough time with the intrathecal chemo yesterday, I slept better last night than I have in a long time. I fell asleep around 10:30, and woke up as usual between 2 and 3 am, but I listened to Carole King's "Music," which struck me as incredibly rich and melodious. I fell back asleep until after 7. Then I got up, showered, and was ready when Emma awoke.

Emma was wearing a grey and white striped shirt and ripped jeans. I had on a skirt and blue shirt, and wore a brown hat we picked up at Bloomingdale's last week. We buzzed for a cab and our favorite car service driver, Mischa, was there. He's a Russian immigrant who enjoys practicing his English—every time we drive with him he has incorporated some new big word into his vocabulary. He drove us to Christine's.

We took the small elevator up, and there were white halls with white doors, each one a different place of business. When we knocked on Christine's door, a young woman answered who said she was Christine's assistant. Jen, the place was perfect. Her studio was small, about the size of the first office I ever had at the hospital, with hardwood floors and white walls. All around us were a million wall hooks and hat stands, and every available space was covered with hats. There were all the hats I had seen on line and even a few more hats that are for her new spring collection. The hats were in every color of the rainbow, in every possible style and a million different fabrics. I said to Emma, "Oh, Emma, we've come to the right place."

Christine entered. She was about my age, long dark straight hair, tall, nice smile. She told us that she was inspired to go into the hat business by her love for the theater when she was young. Christine also said that people talk to people who wear hats. I said, "That's good, because I want people to talk to me!" and she said "Me too!" We turned our full attention to the hats.

I tried on hat after hat. I had studied the hats online and knew a lot of their names, which impressed Christine. I tried on some of the hats I recognized and others that I hadn't seen. The hats differed in the crown (shape of the top), material (straw or fabric, including silk, cotton, a fine weave, satin, or a sort of rain-proof material), brim size (small, medium, large), brim direction (neutral, up, or down), and trim (band, bow, flowers, feathers, combination, or none). Some hats sat higher on the head than others; after I lose my hair, the ones that sit lower will be better.

I tried on the Easy and the Davenport and the Roz and the Natasha and the Reese Paisley and the Lucy and the Ruby and the Butterfly, and some cotton hats whose names I don't remember, and the Lachlan and I don't even know what else. Turquoise and rust and brown and black and tan and white and pink and gray. Across the room, I spotted a hat in a beautiful shade of purple with a big flower. I had to get that one. I said to Christine, "With a hat like that, I have to win."

By the end, I had ordered 15 hats! After we paid, Christine asked if she should ship them, and I said yes. She's shipping them on Monday; they should arrive on Tuesday. When Emma is in Paris on Tuesday, she will know that somewhere in New York I am getting a huge delivery of beautiful birthday hats in huge white hat boxes tied up with big yellow satin ribbons.

At the end, I gave Christine a big hug and she asked me what kind of cancer I have. I told her it was lymphoma. She asked how far along I was in the treatment. I replied that I'd had neurosurgery already, and had received three of 18 chemo treatments.

I got the hats for a lot of reasons. I did it because I like to look for silver linings. I did it to teach Emma that even when life is hard, you can do things to make it better. I did it because it gave me something wonderful to think about for the past few days as I started chemo. And I did it because it will help me beat this. Because honestly, Jen, how can I lose the battle with cancer if I'm wearing a hat like that?

Love
Laura

From: Laura
Sent: Friday, March 23, 2007 3:19 PM
To: Cindy
Subject: Balloons!

Hi Cindy and "Breast Friends" (Cindy, can you forward this to all co-conspirators?)!

I'm writing to thank you for the incredible bunch of pink balloons that you sent. I have never seen so many balloons in one place. They are a fabulously happy birthday present, and will be even more therapeutic than the chemo. Thanks!

Love
Laura

From: Laura
Sent: Saturday, March 24, 2007 4:23 AM
To: Jennifer
Subject: Birthday balloons

Hi Jen. Happy birthday to me! Yesterday after Emma and I got home from the hat shopping, we were resting in the family room and the doorman buzzed, and came up with a huge bouquet of balloons in different shades of pink, all helium-filled, with long twisty pink ribbons that came together tied to a weight with a pretty bow at the bottom. The balloons (which were from the "Balloon Salloon," I kid you not) could barely fit through our front door! The gift was from Cindy and the other breast folks. They had wanted to throw me a party on Monday but I wasn't up for it—the balloons were the perfect birthday gift. Emma and I laughed, and even the boys laughed about it when they got home.

Emma is going to Paris today for spring break, and David has been working hard to get everything ready for her. He also had to do our taxes, and is dealing with legal stuff for us. The kids were both out for awhile last night with friends, so David and I had a little time together. We sat and listened to Bill Evans and made a list of things to do, and then we curled up to watch the Hitchcock movie with Cary Grant and Grace Kelly, To Catch a Thief.

Keep writing. What music are you playing now?

Love
Laura

From: Laura
Sent: Saturday, March 24, 2007 9:38 PM
To: Jennifer
Subject: Birthday

Hi Jen. Thanks for the wonderful Blue Mountain birthday card! And that's terrific that you're working on the Bach Suites for Unaccompanied Cello. I have a recording of Yo-Yo Ma playing them on my iPod, and it's one of my

favorites—especially the first part (prelude) of Suite 1 in G
Major.

I had a fabulous 47th birthday. I went back to sleep after
I wrote to you, and I felt good when I woke up. It was beautiful
here, sunny and just a little cool. Emma woke up first. I
snuggled with her in bed and she told me about a party she went
to with her friends last night. David woke up and we awakened
Nate, who likes to be at the soup kitchen where he volunteers by
10 am. We all had breakfast together—David made scrambled
eggs and home fries. Thank God Emma inherited her cooking
talent from David, not from me. When we were in college, I
was a better cook than David, but then he met a guy in his
medical school class who was a gourmet chef on the side and
taught David everything he knew.

Today, to celebrate my birthday, we separated the pink
balloons from their attached weight so that the balloons could
fly all over the apartment. We played an impromptu game of
balloon volley ball, and David and the kids let me win, because
I'm the birthday girl. Emma tied four balloons to the glass at the
top of the walls on our terrace. They look festive, especially
since it's a little windy and the balloons are dancing in the
breeze.

The family did the traditional "Showering of the
birthday person with gifts," in which the rest of the family
practically trips over each other to keep a secret of the wrapping
of presents and the signing of cards, and a bag is brought to the
"surprised" guest of honor (who is never quite surprised). They
gave me gifts I'll definitely use: books by Perri Klass, a woman
doctor who is one of my favorite writers, and CDs to put on my
iPod (Glen Gould playing Bach Goldberg Variations, the album
from the Producers, and an amazing jazz guitarist named Nino
Josele playing the music of Bill Evans). Nate went to his

volunteer gig, and Emma and David finished packing for her trip.

David had rented a car to drive Emma to her school today, because the kids going on the class trip were all meeting there to take a bus to JFK for their trip to Paris. I wasn't sure I'd be up for the car ride, about an hour each way, but it was a gorgeous day and I felt good so I went. Emma was the first student there. We met Emma's French teacher, and then Emma took us on a little walk on the beautiful campus and showed us her favorite deli for lunch where they name their sandwiches after superheroes. We were unanimous—we all wanted the Batman, which has turkey, honey mustard, and slices of green apple. After a quick lunch we walked back up the hill to her school, helped Emma get her bag on the bus, and waved goodbye. She went off to Paris.

I finally get the secret of living a good life. You have to create your magic in each individual day. Today, for example, there was the birthday and the balloons and seeing Emma off; yesterday we got the hats; and last weekend we had David's birthday party. There's always a lot of shit that will either be prescheduled or will happen spontaneously. The way to make the balance good is to pack in the good stuff too. I bet that advice is in every self-help book I've ever read and ignored, but somehow I get it now. Even on the days when I have chemo or something else that sucks, I can build some magic into it. Maybe in this book I can express that in a way that will help people understand. You shouldn't have to get Stage IV lymphoma to figure it out.

Got to go. Energy is fading. Nate had a friend over for awhile and they watched March madness (college basketball) on TV. Since UCLA beat Kansas, Nate is leading his NCAA bracket now. Life is sweet.

Love
Laura

From: Laura
Sent: Sunday, March 25, 2007 7:41 AM
To: Emma
Subject: To Paris from New York

Hi Emma. It's Sunday morning and I'm in the living room, writing to you from the lap top. I slept well and feel good. Half the birthday balloons are still as high as the ceiling, and the other half have sunk to about my height. A few are almost on the floor. How many days will it take all of them to come down, I wonder? The balloons that you tied to the terrace walls are still there, dancing in the breeze, but now they are just slightly higher than eye level. I like to see them because they remind me of you.
I love you more than the sun, the moon, and the stars. Can't wait to hear about your trip.

Love
Mom

From: Emma
Sent: Sunday, March 25, 2007 12:34 PM
To: Mom
Subject: From Emma in France

Dear Mom,

There's a computer in the lobby of this hotel that I'm using to write you this email. All the computer commands are in French! I should be able to get back here tomorrow, but I'm not sure, and I have no idea whether or not the hotel in Paris has a computer. The flight was good. I slept on the plane for a few hours. Tell Dad that bringing extra contacts was a brilliant idea because I could take them out before I fell asleep and put new ones in when I woke up.

After we got off the plane, we went to a part of town where we walked around, shopped, and ate. I had a brie, tomato, and watercress sandwich on baguette and a waffle with bananas and chocolate. I also took a lot of amazing pictures and I'm worried that I might not have enough space on my camera if I keep taking around 250 pictures a day.

Sun Moon Stars
Love
Emma

From: Laura
Sent: Sunday, March 25, 2007 4:47 PM
To: Emma
Subject: Love to Emma in Paris

Dearest Emma,

Thanks for your email! Now you understand how I used to feel when I was traveling a lot for work, and my biggest challenge of each day on the road was to figure out how to get to the next computer so that I could send and check email. Don't worry, I'll assume it may be days before you get to check it; if there's anything urgent, Dad and I can get in touch with you through your French teacher.

It's still a beautiful Sunday. Dad was out for most of the morning to round on his patients at the hospital and then he went grocery shopping. Nate and I talked about a short story he's reading for English by Melville called Bartleby the Scrivener, about a man named Bartleby who works as a "scribe" or copyist for a lawyer, and whenever anyone asks him to do anything, he says, "I would prefer not." Nate has to write a paper about it, so that's what he's doing today.

I love that you're taking so many pictures. When we went on our family trip to Paris a few years ago for Aunt Laura's "end of chemo celebration tour," I took a million digital pictures too—do you remember? I had to spend hours downloading them each day so I would have enough memory on the camera to take more pictures the next day! Thank goodness for those electrical adapters.

I'm so glad Elena is your roommate. I know you hoped she would be. And I really love her parents—they're always so nice at school events, and I liked talking to them at your recent basketball game.

I've been listening to French music in honor of your being in Paris. There's a beautiful sonata for clarinet and piano by a Parisian composer named Poulenc that I used to play in chamber music class with my friend Susan, who was a wonderful clarinetist. The sonata has three movements: allegro tristamente (fast and sadly), romanza tres calme (romantic and very calm), and allegro con fuoco, tres anime (fast with fire, very animated). We can listen to it together when you get home.

G2G (see? I listened when you taught me that G2G means Got To Go). Going to take a nap. I love you so much.

Sun Moon Stars
Love
Mom

From: Laura
Sent: Tuesday, March 27, 2007 1:07 AM
To: Jennifer
Subject: Liberation

Hi Jen. Don't worry that you and Sophie had to interrupt your shopping because she was fussing. It's OK that Sophie is not an Olympic shopper yet. Emma took awhile to grow into her profound love of shopping, and now she is everything I could have dreamed of in a shopping companion and more.

Monday was fine. I went to the office. Cindy organized a birthday lunch for me with all the techs—chicken vegetable soup and vanilla frozen yogurt, two of my favorite foods. I went home to Nate by 4 pm, and we made a game of guessing how many days it would take for all of the balloons to fall down. The person who guesses closest without going over is the winner— no prizes, just the satisfaction of success. Some of those balloons are still hanging up there by the ceiling! The ones that fall we either throw away, puncture, or "liberate"—we go onto the terrace and release the balloons into the sky. The balloon liberation was Nate's idea—at first I was going to discourage this practice because I was concerned about its impact on global warming, but then I thought hey, it looks like fun

Love
Laura

From: Laura
Sent: Tuesday, March 27, 11:26 PM
To: Jennifer
Subject: Cornell trip

Dearest Jen,

Let me tell you about this amazing adventure Nate & I had today. Last week we had to fill out some forms for Nate's college applications, and on one of the questions they asked if we had any personal ties to specific colleges. David and I wrote about where we went, but then Nate asked me, "Mom, aren't you a professor at Cornell or something?" and I realized that yes, I am! Along with my faculty appointment at Memorial, I have a medical school appointment at the Weill Medical College of Cornell University. Here I am, always advising the women faculty to be aware of all of their appointments, and I don't even remember my own! That got Nate thinking about Cornell.

We planned a day trip to visit Cornell. It had to be today. Tomorrow (Wednesday) I get intrathecal chemo at 3 pm and Thursday I'm admitted for inpatient chemo, so this is my narrow window. We arranged to take a flight from LaGuardia to Ithaca that was supposed to take off at 8:30 am and land at 10 am. We planned to take a tour at either 11 am or 1 pm depending on exactly when we get in and stroll around the campus. I also booked a hotel for the day (they have a hotel school at Cornell, so they actually have a real hotel called the Statler right on campus) so that if I get sick or tired I could sleep. We booked the return flight for that evening from Ithaca to LaGuardia.

The day deviated from the plan. We got on our flight, but the plane sat on the runway for 45 minutes before it took off, and then they couldn't land in Ithaca because of fog. We circled in the sky for over an hour, and finally they landed in Syracuse at 11 am. So much for the 11 am tour. By the time we got to the Cornell Admissions Office in Ithaca, it was 1:15 pm, and the 1 pm tour had already left. Nate and I were both tired and hungry by then, so I suggested that we just go to the hotel, dump our stuff, have lunch, and explore the campus ourselves.

The Statler Hotel was right next door to the admissions office, and it was like a quaint country inn. I had booked a room on the 9th floor with twin beds so we could both lie down if necessary and have our own space. Jen, the view of the campus and mountains from that 9th floor window was breathtaking. It was worth the whole trip just to see that view. Nate and I pulled up two chairs to the window and looked at the map of Cornell, and Nate figured out which building was which. We ordered room service for lunch. I got tired after lunch and took a nap while Nate went off to explore on his own.

When I woke up two hours later at 4:00, the sun had come out. The first thing I saw was the panoramic view of the campus, including an old clock tower with bells that chime like a European cathedral every 15 minutes. I got up and splashed some water on my face and at that moment, Nate walked in. He had explored and procured us ice water and fresh fruit. I asked him to take me on a tour, and he gave me the short version: two stops and three breaks. We went to the James Olin library and the Cornell store, and Nate bought Cornell t-shirts for the whole family. After a quick dinner at the hotel, we went back to the Ithaca airport and took an uneventful trip home.

The trip meant a lot to me. I was touched by the way Nate looked out for me. It was great to imagine him in that pastoral setting and to see his life opening up with possibilities.

I liked helping him get familiar with the process of the college visit, so he can make some future visits on his own or with friends. Best of all, I loved the fact that we seized the moment between two chemos to do something special. I've since found out that my white blood cell count was essentially zero when I went. Breathing recirculated plane air is not a great idea when you have no white blood cells with which to fight infection, so I'm glad I didn't know my white blood cell count at the time—I probably would have been scared to go, and I would have missed it.

Got to go to sleep—out of juice. More tomorrow.

Love
Laura

From: Laura
Sent: Wednesday, March 28, 2007 7:30 AM
To: Jennifer
Subject: Third time's a charm

Hi Jen. Great news. You know how I've been vomiting like crazy every time they give me the intrathecal methotrexate? Well, today I didn't throw up!

I was scheduled for my third dose at 3 pm. I had been taking a nap, and I forgot to ask Carmen to wake me up, so I almost overslept my doctor's appointment. Luckily I had arranged to meet Cindy at the oncologist's before 3. Thank God for Cindy—when she couldn't find me, she called me on my cell phone. I was the last appointment of the day, but Cindy convinced them to stay to give me the chemo. Good thing I only live ten blocks from the hospital. I jumped in a cab to Memorial.

This time, the intrathecal methotrexate was much better. As Phil had suggested last week, I took some anti-nausea meds beforehand. There is a wonderful pill called Zofran that tastes sweet and melts in your mouth—which is perfect, because when you're nauseated, you don't really feel like swallowing anything. Unfortunately, Zofran costs about $40 per pill. Remember the episode of Seinfeld where Elaine is worried that the Today Sponge, her favorite form of contraception, may be discontinued? She buys a case of Sponges, which may be the last in existence, and before having sex with a guy, she has to decide if he's "spongeworthy." Well, when I'm nauseated, I have to decide if the nausea is "Zofran-worthy" or if one of the many cheaper nausea pills (like Compazine) would work. Intrathecal chemo is definitely Zofran-worthy.

When Phil came in to give the intrathecal injection, Cindy jumped up to spray my head. Phil had trouble getting the needle into the Omaya, and encountered a fair amount of resistance to injection, so he had to inject very slowly. An injection that usually takes seconds now took a couple of minutes. I waited for the nausea, but it never came. I felt so fine that I asked Phil afterwards, "Are you sure you gave me the chemo?" Yes, he was. Maybe it was the Zofran, but I wonder whether the injection rate also has something to do with it. Could it be that a slower injection of intrathecal chemo is less likely to cause nausea and vomiting? I have to ask Sam, my neurologist.

First admission tomorrow. I'll write from "inside the house."

Love
Laura

From: Laura
Sent: Wednesday, March 28, 2007 9:35 PM
To: Cindy
Subject: Thanks, and hats

Hi Cindy. Thanks for calling me today to wake me up to get chemo, and for making them stay to give it to me.
And guess what? The hats came!

Love
Laura

Chapter 6
First Admission

Get doctors you trust, and listen to their advice.

From: Laura
Sent: Thursday, March 29, 2007 11:59 PM
To: Nate
Subject: Your visit

Hi Nate. Thanks so much for coming to visit me on my first evening in the hospital. I take it as a good sign that there was a 5-episode marathon of The Office on TV.

I'm delighted about the SAT. What a relief to know that you're done with that now. It's a huge weight off your shoulders, and one that you've been carrying around for months. Let it feel lighter—it is!

The college thing will sort itself out. It's great that you're figuring out what you want in a school. You'll have a lot more information about all the schools by the time you make a choice.

Tomorrow is Dad's actual 50th birthday—can you make sure to wish him a happy birthday from me first thing in the morning, and give my love to Emma?

I love you, Nate.

Love
Mom

From: Laura
Sent: Friday, March 30, 2007 12:49 AM
To: Jennifer
Subject: First hospital admission

Hi Jen. It was so wonderful of you to call and wish me luck the night before I was admitted. I was a little nervous about being hospitalized. I thought I was acting pretty cool about the whole thing, but you can see right through me, as usual. It just shows your insight into the human psyche (or at least into mine!). I like your suggestion that if I'm scared, I should just listen to Bach.

Let me tell you today's chemo story. We got in at 9 am Thursday morning to admitting, and a woman named Sandy checked me in. We were supposed to wait for Escort but they took forever—now there's a shock!—so David and I jumped ship and went up to the eighth floor ourselves (I promised the woman in admitting that we would claim we snuck out and would never let on that she knew we were leaving). David helped me settle into the room here. We put my iPod and cell phone on a little table beside the bed, on their respective chargers. The room had a bed on which I spread a fuzzy green blanket from home, window with view, TV, DVD player, closet, private bathroom, and working hospital computer. I take the computer as definitive proof of the existence of God.

The floor I'm on, M8, is the Bone Marrow Transplant (BMT) floor. Although I'm not getting a BMT now (that's plan B if the chemo is unsuccessful), sometimes lymphoma patients who are not getting transplants stay on this floor. Every patient gets a single room for two reasons. First, BMT patients are susceptible to infection, so they like to keep them isolated.

Second, because the BMT patients are often here for long periods of time, sometimes up to two months or longer, most of the rooms are spacious enough that a family member can sleep over. Another thing that's good about being here is that if I do end up needing a BMT eventually, at least I'll be familiar with where it's going to happen.

The nurse, Trish, accessed the port, which she did fairly painlessly, using the spray. We started with four hours of hydration using a salt solution (normal saline with bicarbonate), with the goal of making the urine less acidic and more alkaline so that the methotrexate won't crystallize in the kidneys. They check the urine pH, which is a measure of acidity, before giving the methotrexate—the higher the pH, the less acidic and the more alkaline, and you want the urine to be alkaline, meaning a pH of 7.5 or higher. Mine was 8 (I've always been an overachiever). When the urine is alkalinized, they run in the methotrexate, a large bag of ugly yellow stuff.

One of the main complications of the methotrexate is painful ulcers in your gastrointestinal tract anywhere from the mouth (north) to the derriere (south). Trish told me that the best way to prevent those ulcers was by rinsing my mouth out frequently with a mouthwash called Biotene or with a bicarbonate wash. I did that every hour while I was awake.

The night nurse, Jonathan, was very nice and knew what he was doing. I had no problems or reactions, and I've been peeing up a storm—the goal is 150 cc/hr and I am doing far better. They'll hydrate me more tonight and check another urine pH. If the pH is too low, meaning it's acidic, I'll need to take oral bicarbonate.

Aimee, the ultrasound technologist from 64th Street, came to visit today with a card about how the Lord is walking by my side. When people ask what they can do to help, I say without hesitation, "Pray for me." I can't tell you how comforting it is to have people from all different religions praying for me. I have Jews writing my name on a piece of paper and sticking it in the Wailing Wall in Jerusalem and former radiology trainees in Croatia making pilgrimages. A dear friend of mine in New Orleans sent me a small wooden bracelet with pictures of the saints. I grew up in a reformed Jewish household and was never much of a believer, but somehow I feel that this positive energy in the universe channeled in my direction has got to help. And maybe there's more out there than we think.

I love you very much. I know you will have an incredible son. It is so great to have a boy and a girl!

Love
Laura

From: Laura
Sent: Friday, March 30, 2007 1:19 AM
To: David
Subject: Happy Birthday!

Dearest David,
(Imagine wild music in the background and a strip tease)
Happy birthday to you
Happy birthday to you
Happy birthday dear David
Happy birthday to you
Are you 1, 2, 3, 4, 5, 6, 7, 8, 9, 10, 11, 12, 13, 14, 15, 16, 17, 18, 19, 20, 21, 22, 23, 24, 25, 26, 27, 28, 29, 30, 31, 32, 33, 34, 35, 36, 37, 38, 39, 40, 41, 42, 43, 44, 45, 46, 47, 48, 49, 50?

(You can't be 50; to me we will always be college students, making love in a carrel in Baker library.)

I think our boy and girl will both be OK. I love you today and every day.

Love
Laura

From: Laura
Sent: Friday, March 30, 2007 2:23 AM
To: Sam
Subject: Update, and question

Hi Sam. Just an update and a question. I tolerated the first IV R-CHOP without a hitch. I've had three courses of the intrathecal methotrexate. My first two intrathecal chemos were injected fast and I puked my guts out, but the third was injected much more slowly and it went fine. Does injecting the intrathecal chemo slowly decrease the likelihood of nausea and vomiting?

Best wishes
Laura

From: Laura
Sent: Friday, March 30, 2007 2:37 AM
To: Cindy
Subject: St. Patrick's cathedral

Hi Cindy. Can I come with you one day soon to St. Patrick's cathedral, where you've been lighting candles? I've never been. Maybe one day next week?

Am I allowed to light a candle for myself, or is that considered "self-referral"? ☺

Love
Laura

From: Laura
Sent: Saturday, March 31, 2007 1:23 AM
To: Jennifer
Subject: More stories from inside

Hi Jen. Another day, and so many stories. I can't believe I was just admitted two days ago—it feels like a lifetime has gone by.

This morning there was a risk management lecture in the Department of Medicine Grand Rounds in Hoffman from 8-9 am. The Departmental secretary had emailed us that we should try to go to this one if possible; otherwise the Radiology one is in August, which is pretty far away. So I asked permission to go to the lecture, which was an elevator ride downstairs from M8. The doc covering the lymphoma service said it was OK, so I went with face mask, IV pole, and all. It was funny how people responded—most people already seemed to know; some looked right through me; and some were terrific, as I would have expected. I sat with a couple of friends from Radiology. The lecture wasn't great. A malpractice lawyer spoke, and she was disorganized and didn't say much. But it was good to get off the floor for awhile.

Did you know that when you're an inpatient at Memorial, you're entitled to a massage from Integrative Medicine? I had Reflexology, which is a massage for your hands and feet. If the computer in the room didn't convince me of Divine Intervention, the Reflexology did. If it weren't for the chemo, my room would be a prime vacation spot!

David and Nate came to see me yesterday. It was David's 50th birthday; he looked exhausted. Nate was in a good mood. I think he feels better about applying to college now that he's visited a school. Even if he decides not to apply to Cornell, our trip there seems to have demystified the process. I had other visitors yesterday also, including Cindy, who brought me frozen yogurt.

I'm not sleeping much, but I'm getting a lot of writing done. Sam agrees that the third intrathecal methotrexate was easier than the first two because the oncologist injected it very slowly the third time. Apparently, when you inject it too fast, once the chemo hits the fourth ventricle it tickles the vomiting center in your brain and you puke. I'm going to ask the oncologist to inject it more slowly in the future.

Looks like they're shooting for a possible Monday discharge, but it depends on the methotrexate level. As Phil said, "It's all about urination now." I have been exceeding expectations in the urine output department. They want 150 cc/hr. I laugh at their 150 cc/hr, and raise it by 50 cc/hr!!

Thanks for the Bach suggestion. I listened on the iPod not only to Yo-Yo Ma playing the Bach Unaccompanied Cello Suite in G Major (one of my favorite pieces of all time), but also to the other five unaccompanied cello suites, to Hilary Hahn playing Bach partitas for solo violin, and to Glenn Gould playing the Bach Two- and Three-Part Inventions. You're right—Bach has a way of making order and beauty out of turbulence and chaos.

Love
Laura

From: Laura
Sent: Saturday, March 31, 2007 6:07 AM
To: Jennifer
Subject: Saturday morning

Hi J—Saturday morning, almost 6 o'clock. Didn't sleep much last night. The chemo part is done; the rest is just the leucovorin "chaser" and fluids. That will help lower the methotrexate level until it's low enough that it's safe to go home.

My hats arrived at the house last week (not a moment too soon), but in the hospital I've just been wearing the Monk cap that Cindy gave me. I can't believe how Cindy has been there for me during my treatment. What a silver lining.

Charlie, who works in the file room of our outpatient breast center, is going to visit me today and bring home-made soup. He is a fantastic cook. When I was a resident taking weekend call and Charlie worked in the file room at the hospital, he used to bring in these savory lunches he had cooked with rice and chicken and shrimp and some kind of soup with a tomato base and a secret combination of spices. He also used to bring in fresh salad with these amazing tomatoes that he grew in his garden. All of the residents wanted to work on the weekends when Charlie was there.

Emma gets home from Paris today and will come to see me tomorrow. I can't wait to see her and hear about her trip.

Got to go—they want another urine sample. There's a Murphy's law (you know, "whatever can go wrong, will") that says the nurses' aide always dumps the urine before they get to send it to the lab. I'm swigging the Gatorade now.

Love
Laura

From: Laura
Sent: Sunday, April 1, 2007 1:44 AM
To: Jennifer
Subject: Hair

Hi Jen. David picked Emma up at the Newark Airport last night, and I get to see her later today.

My hair is falling out. It's so bizarre. You know how you brush your hair, and when you get to the bottom it stops? Well, now it just keeps going, and all the hair comes out in the brush. I know a lot of women who shaved their heads when that started happening, but I cling to the hope that a curl or two will hang on for dear life. Oh well, hair grows back. David said to me, "In September, the cancer will be gone, and so will your hair, and I couldn't care less about the hair."

Nate also helped me feel better about losing my hair. One of our family's favorite TV shows is West Wing, the Sorkin drama about a fictitious Democratic President named Josiah Bartlett and his White House staffers. Early in the campaign, Bartlett keeps asking, "What's next?" The staffers ask Leo, Bartlett's close friend and future Chief of Staff, what Bartlett means by that. Leo explains that Bartlett is saying that he understands the situation, has dealt with it, and is ready to move on. Nate reassured me that losing my hair means that the chemo is working, and that hair grows back. He added, "It's OK,

Mom. You can handle it. Do what Bartlett would do. Just ask, what's next?"

Love
Laura

From: Laura
Sent: Sunday, April 1, 2007 7:49 PM
To: Jennifer
Subject: Laps and family visits

Dearest Jen,

Today was a wonderful day. After I emailed you, I put on my shoes and a mask and went strolling multiple laps around the nurses' station with my IV pole. The only problem with doing laps is that I have to unplug the IV pole from the wall to do it, and since the batteries are low the pump starts beeping and you have to hit "silence" every couple of minutes. But that's a small price to pay for the freedom to roam.

The bone marrow transplant patients on this floor often aren't allowed to leave their rooms. It's such a luxury to be able to walk around. M8 was recently redecorated; the hallway walls are covered with large nature photos of trees, flowers, different seasons, sun, snow, and birds in the sky. The pictures (selected by Holly, the floor's wonderful Nurse Manager) make you feel like there are windows looking out on a rustic landscape. There is also a small room called the family pantry where they have a fridge and freezer that patients and their families can use. They have coffee, tea, water, and juice there too. This morning I "went out for breakfast"—I lapped around the nurses' station and went to the family pantry and had some delicious decaf with skim milk.

David and Emma came in the early afternoon. Emma was wearing a stunning pair of turquoise shoes that she bought on the street in Paris. They were perfect on her—they even showed toe cleavage (this is the latest thing—what a term!). She bought me a necklace with an antique chain and stones in muted colors as well as a little card from Paris with a hand-painted picture of a Parisian café. I have a bulletin board with tacks in my room, and she wrote "Emma" in the tacks on the bulletin board. David and Emma stayed about an hour and a half, and Emma told us all about her trip. After they left, I liked looking at the bulletin board, and seeing the "Emma" design—it made me feel like she was still there.

Nate came later. We had a quiet visit. Sometimes we didn't talk; I just read the paper while he was surfing the net on the computer. We walked 7 laps around the nurses' station together before he went home.

The Op Ed page of the Sunday Times featured a piece by Dr. Harold Varmus, the Nobel prize-winning scientist who is the President of Memorial, in which he said that we are winning the war against cancer. I always wanted to win the war on cancer, but for some reason I'm particularly passionate about it now.

Love
Laura

From: Laura
Sent: Monday, April 2, 2007 12:10 AM
To: Nate
Subject: Fro yo

Hi Nate. Thank you for coming to visit me, and bringing the frozen yogurt ("fro yo")! I just took my midnight "constitutional" and got some fro yo in the family pantry—I finished the one that was almost empty and got a good healthy start on the one you brought. Thanks for providing my midnight snack. Now I'm listening to Stevie Wonder singing "Ribbon in the Sky," another beautiful song. I only did another one lap instead of seven more this evening, but it was good.
    Love to Dad and Emma.

Love
Mom

From: Laura
Sent: Monday, April 2, 2007 1:36 AM
To: Frances
Subject: Prayer group

Hi Frances. Please thank your prayer group for the beautiful prayer they sent me, called "I Asked God."

I asked God to take away my pain. God said, No.
It is not for me to take away, but for you to give it up.
I asked God to make my handicapped child whole. God said, No.
His spirit is whole, his body is only temporary.
I asked God to grant me patience. God said, No.
Patience is a byproduct of tribulations; it isn't granted, it is learned.
I asked God to give me happiness. God said, No.
I give you blessings. Happiness is up to you.
I asked God to spare me pain. God said, No.
Suffering draws you apart from worldly cares and brings you
       closer to Me.
I asked God to make my spirit grow. God said, No.
You must grow on your own, but I will prune you to make you
       fruitful.
I asked God for all things that I might enjoy life. God said, No.
I gave you life, so that you may enjoy all things.
I asked God to help me love others, as much as He loves me.
God said Ahhhh, finally you have the idea.

Love
Laura

From: Laura
Sent: Monday, April 2, 2007 7:21 AM
To: David
Subject: Coming home

    Hi Babe. Just a note to thank you for bringing your button-down green flannel shirt for me to wear this morning. It makes me feel protected by you. It's much easier to maneuver a button-down shirt than a pullover shirt when I'm hooked up to an IV—to get out of the pullover, I actually have to push it down to the floor and step out of it, and step into the next shirt and pull it up. And there's another advantage to the button-down—it has a pocket for me to put the iPod in! I walked multiple laps around the nurses' station this morning and then "went out for coffee" to the Family Pantry. Apparently 14 laps is a mile (a patient on 12 clocked it), so I can even quantify my exercise—I walked more than a mile today!

I slept well last night and took a good shower this morning. They're still giving me the leukovorin "rescue." It's my favorite part of the chemo. I'd much rather have someone give me a "rescue" than a "CHOP." They really have to rethink the names of these chemo regimens—"CHOP" is bad enough, but apparently there's another one called "ICE." What kind of message does that send? Anyway, I just called the cafeteria (euphemistically referred to as "room service") to order breakfast, and they picked up the phone right away. Scrambled eggs and toast and decaf and a fresh orange and a banana.

They run the methotrexate level at noon, so it probably won't be back until 2. Do you want me to call you when they are actually discharging me? It'll probably be sometime between 2 and 5 pm. I really want to go home today, so before they take my temperature, I will suck on ice chips to make sure there is no fever (only kidding—although it's tempting).

I got an email from a former Croatian breast imaging trainee. He told me to "beat that crazy lymphocyte!"

I love you.

Love
Laura

Chapter 7
Home

Cancer is the best excuse you'll ever have—use it!

From: Laura
Sent: Monday, April 2, 2007 10:00 PM
To: Jennifer
Subject: Home

Hi J. I am home, and it is even more wonderful than I remembered. Just to be free from the IV pole is bliss.

Hope your Seder was fun. Did you drink in the reclining position? Who asked the 4 questions? Sophie's probably too young, or maybe her questions were, "When do we eat? Can we eat now? When can we play? When do we go home?"

Happy Passover.

Love
Laura

From: Laura
Sent: Tuesday, April 3, 2007 10:56 PM
To: Jennifer
Subject: Shopping with Emma

Dearest Jen,

Emma and I went on a shopping spree today after work to get spring clothes. I wore one of my Christine Moore hats for the first time. I chose the Easy, which has a beige straw cloth slouch crown with a medium up brim, a little bow, and thin trim in a pattern of tiny vertical stripes in turquoise, pink, yellow, and white.

First, we went to a shoe store called Arche. They had just gotten in their spring sandals, and they had a style that fit me perfectly: it was as if they had custom designed these shoes for my feet! I bought them in four colors (turquoise, yellow, pink, and tan). We went to Eileen Fisher, and I bought some clothes to wear when I'm in the hospital. Then we went to Olive & Bette's to get summer camp clothes for Emma. David thinks I was having a manic episode, and maybe I was, but losing your hair is tough—I had no idea my head was so white—and the stuff I got will help me feel beautiful, or at least I'll feel like my shoes and clothes are beautiful.

Tomorrow I'm going to work in the Women's Office. Thursday I have to get a blood test, and then I'm going back to the wig place. Now I wish I'd just gotten a wig with short hair. Life is too short to waste time with stuff that doesn't matter.

Love
Laura

From: Laura
Sent: Thursday, April 5, 2007 5:22 AM
To: Cindy
Subject: Re: checking on you

Hi Cindy! I missed you yesterday too!
I came to work and got great stuff done in the Women's Office. Did I tell you I'd like to create a Women's Oncology

Network (abbreviated WON) that is an international society of women doctors and scientists dedicated to eradicating cancer? So yesterday, I decided on the T-shirt slogan, and on the society stone and color.

Here's an excerpt from the grant proposal.

****

The goal of WON is to provide mentorship, collaboration, and unity among women physicians and scientists dedicated to the clinical treatment and research investigation of cancer. Our T-shirt slogan will be: "WON for all and all for WON!"

The color/stone of WON will be turquoise, long considered a stone that is holy, brings good fortune, and fends off the evil eye. Al Qazwini, the Persian scholar, wrote: "The hand that wears a turquoise and seals with it will never know poverty." The Aztecs in Mexico believed that the sky blue gemstone directly connects the sky and the sea. In Orthodox Judaism, turquoise is the only non-white thread in the prayer shawl, representing the uniqueness of individuals. Turquoise has been deemed to provide protection from darkness, to guard horses and riders from unexpected falls, to endow shy people with confidence, and to be responsible for faithfulness and constancy in relationships. Turquoise is the perfect stone for WON.

****

Between you and me, the real reason I picked turquoise is because I love that color and it goes with my eyes. I'm also tired of pink for girls and blue for boys. This way we get our own blue, and a beautiful blue it is!I stopped by to see you in Mammo but it was after 5 pm and I must have just missed you.

I wanted to show you my new hat, called the Natasha. It's a soft weave with a medium brim, silk binding, and a beautiful silk bow, all in a deep violet.

Love
Laura

From: Laura
Sent: Sunday, April 8, 2007 8:56 PM
To: Jennifer
Subject: Quiet Sunday

Dearest Jen,
       Today was quiet. I went out for a walk in the sun, but came home after a block and a freezing gust of wind. A good day to stay home and be warm. Emma and I watched the DVD of Season 1 of Project Runway (one of our favorite shows). Now I'm going to bed.

Love
Laura

From: Laura
Sent: Monday, April 9, 2007 9:57 PM
To: Jennifer
Subject: Playing the cancer card

Dearest Jen,

My friend Maureen taught me that cancer is the best excuse you'll ever have, so use it—she calls it "playing the cancer card." So far I've only done it once, to get the dinner reservations for David's birthday party. But today I found the perfect opportunity to do it again.

In our building, people generally get cabs on a first-come, first-served basis. But you know how some people believe that the social contract doesn't apply to them? Well, there is one Evil Woman in the building who always jumps the line. It's so annoying—no matter how long you've been waiting, she cuts ahead and barrels into the cab.

Today, I was waiting for a cab when finally it pulled up into the driveway. Suddenly, the Evil Woman appeared and started to cut ahead of me in line. I said to her calmly, "Excuse me, but I have cancer, I need to get chemo, and that's my cab." She stopped in her tracks and stared at me, open-mouthed. While she gaped, I jumped in the cab and drove away. Success! I wish I had thought of doing this a decade ago. And the best part of all—I wasn't even going to chemo, I was going shopping at Bloomingdale's!

Love
Laura

From: Laura
Sent: Tuesday, April 10, 2007 6:19 AM
To: Jimmie
Subject: Statistics, and update

Hi Jimmie. Thanks for the wonderful talk—it's great to be able to discuss how it feels to be a doctor and a cancer patient with the former Chair of Psychiatry at Memorial, who practically invented the field of Psycho-Oncology.

I'd love to read the Steven Gould essay you suggested about statistics in cancer. Now is a perfect time for me to read it, because the statistics are against me. I'd also love to read your book on The Human Side of Cancer. You can send them to me either at the hospital or my home address.

Re update—I'm doing great. I've finished one month out of 6 months of chemo, and I'm a little euphoric about it. I have bought 15 beautiful new hats (I am looking at this not as losing my hair, but as an opportunity to buy new hats), and people are starting to give me hats as presents. I knew that the hats would be a fun distraction for me and would help me feel better during treatment. What I didn't anticipate is another huge benefit: hats are terrific icebreakers. You know how some people just don't know what to say when you have cancer? Well, when somebody can't think of anything to say, I can always ask, "Do you like my hat?" and, relieved, they comment on my hat.

I'm writing a book. I'll send it to you when it's done.

Love
Laura

From: Laura
Sent: Tuesday, April 10, 2007 5:30 PM
To: Jennifer
Subject: Chemo OK today!

Hi Jen. Thanks for the beautiful baseball cap that says "Chemo means never having to have a bad hair day!"

I went for outpatient chemo today. I got to the hospital around 9 am. After my blood test came back, I had to wait two hours for them to mix the R-CHOP so I went to a colleague's office and worked on the computer for awhile. Around 11:30, they started the chemo. Some of the premedications made me sleepy. My nurse was named Marina, from the Ukraine. I got the chemo, napped an hour, and was done by 3:00. It was much quicker than last time—they go slow for the first R-CHOP to make sure you're not going to have a reaction, and since I passed that test, they could go much faster. Tentatively, they plan to admit me to the hospital for another inpatient chemo in two weeks.

I'm sorry you've reached the "no sleep" stage of advanced pregnancy. Do you have funky pillows in many shapes? That seemed to help me. Although being able to breathe probably would also be a big plus. Don't worry, these days will pass, and soon you'll get to meet your wonderful son, and I hope he brings you all the joy that Emma and Nate bring to me.

Love
Laura

From: Laura
Sent: Tuesday, April 10, 2007 8:47 PM
To: Jennifer
Subject: Ode to a Neutrophil

Hi Jen. I know I just wrote to you, but there's one more thing I forgot to tell you. I've been going through piles of old papers at home, throwing away massive amounts of stuff. It's always been hard for me to throw things away, but somehow, having cancer makes it clear to me that there are some things that will never be high enough on my radar screen for me to devote time to them, so I've felt freer to jettison old crap.

While sifting through ancient papers, I found a poem that I wrote during my first year of medical school at Columbia College of Physicians & Surgeons (P&S) about the neutrophil, a white blood cell (also called a polymorphonuclear leukocyte or "poly") that fights infection. This topic is particularly dear to me now because chemo lowers my white blood cell count, making me susceptible to infection. The poem describes how the precursor cell, the myeloblast, grows up into a neutrophil, and then experiences the life and death of a hero combating infection in his host. Here it is:

- -

Ode to a Neutrophil by Laura Liberman

Now once there was a myeloblast in bone marrow awaiting
The day when he would grow up and start differentiating.
His mother, a promyelocyte, urged him with voice emphatic,
"Develop! Get some lysosomes! Be metachromatic!"

He was about to do it when a red blood cell nearby
Said, "You'll regret it if you do it, pal." "Regret it? Why?"
The red blood cell explained to him, "If you become a poly
You'll live 2 days in tissues and then die. It would be folly

For one so young, such as yourself, to throw your life away
And live 2 days when you could live 4 months another way.
"Could live 4 months? How could it be? You mean there's
         hope in sight?"
The myeloblast demanded of the young erythrocyte.

"Of course," replied the RBC, for you know very well
You live 120 days if you're a red blood cell."
So saying, the erythrocyte got up and swam away.
The myeloblast thought over what his friend had had to say,

And he resolved to try it. Yes, he would run any risk
In order to transform into a red biconcave disc.
And so, instead of synthesizing many lysosomes
He tried to make just hemoglobin off his polysomes

So he could carry oxygen just like a red blood cell.
The myeloblast then tried to lose his nucleus as well.
His mom, a metamyelocyte, about to be a band,
Said, "What's holding you up, my son? I do not understand.

You should have had those granules inside you long before.
Now, hurry! There's no time to spare! You can't wait
        anymore!"
"But, Mom," replied the myeloblast, "I can't do what you do
'Cause if I do that I'll become a neutrophil like you,

And die after two days of life. But red blood cells live on
So to erythropoietin I must learn to respond!"
His mother, then a neutrophil, said, "Son, give up this game.
The situation's desperate 'cause the tissues are inflamed.

I know there's an infection. I feel it in my lobes.
I know that those bacteria are entering in droves.
And only we can stop them, son. It's true our life has flaws
I know that we must die for it, but we die for a cause."

She turned and left the bone marrow, swam through the
     sinusoid
And gave a last long look at her delinquent little boy.
He thought it over. No, he couldn't selfishly ignore
His duty as a neutrophil as he had done before.

"Longevity is nice," said he, "but I must do what's right,
And so I'll be a polymorphonuclear leukocyte."
And so, our friend the myeloblast gave up his former ways.
He turned into a neutrophil in less than 14 days.

And then he left the bone marrow, swam through the
     circulation,
Diapedesing when he found the site of inflammation.
"The place is full of bugs!" he cried. "Now what am I to
     do?"
A nearby poly said, "Just eat it, get it inside you,

And let your granules do the rest." Our friend then heard
     the moanin'
Of an unlucky bug who had been coated with opsonin.
He hit it with his 2-1 punch until it was digested
Then turned to other bugs with which the tissue was infested.

It was a hard-fought battle, but the polys won the war.
The tissue, once inflamed, became just as it was before.
But yea, alas, our poly was breathing his last breath.
His two-day life was over. He died a martyr's death.

So let us thank the neutrophil, who gives his life to us
Who fights with our bacteria and dies with them in pus.
No choristers will sing for him. For him will toll no bells,
But we will thank the neutrophil, the noblest of the cells.

93

- -

As I recall, when I recited the poem to Dr. John Lindenbaum's hematology class at Columbia P&S, there wasn't a dry eye in the house.

Love
Laura

Chapter 8
Reaching Out

Ask for what you need. Use your experience to help others.

From: Laura
Sent: Tuesday, April 10, 2007 6:20 PM
To: Mel
Subject: Heads up, and Jung-min

Hi Mel. I am writing for three reasons. First, I want to tell you how wonderful it was to see you at the National Institutes of Health breast cancer meeting on ductal carcinoma in situ (DCIS) in January. I loved your presentation of the data on DCIS from your surgical practice. You don't look a day older than you did when we met in Venezuela 15 years ago. It was like old times.

The second reason is that I want to give you a heads up on some stuff going on with me. I was recently diagnosed with an aggressive marginal B zone lymphoma and started six months of chemotherapy in March. So far, I've received 7 of 18 doses of chemo: 2 of 6 outpatient IV R-CHOPS, 4 of 6 outpatient intrathecal methotrexates, and 1 of 6 high-dose IV methotrexates. If all goes well, I'll be done in September.

But the most important reason I'm writing is reason #3. I have the most fabulous fellow on the planet named Jung-min who has been doing research with me for two years. She has applied for the Oncology Fellowship at your hospital to begin July 2008. Since joining me, she has presented an abstract at a national meeting, written a first-author paper in press, and started a second manuscript. In addition, while I've been getting chemo, she has kept up my huge database on image-guided breast biopsy. Jung-min has allowed me to maintain an active research program when it would have otherwise been impossible. I don't know anyone else who could have stepped to the plate the way she did.

Jung-min will be coming out to interview at your hospital soon (I'll send you the exact dates). I'd love for you to speak with her. I know you're not involved with admissions to the Oncology program, but it would be great if she could sit down and talk to you about the pros and cons of the different programs in your area that she's considering, to help her decide what would be best for her.

She can be shy at first, but I know she'll be comfortable with you. Don't let her quiet demeanor dissuade you. Jung-min is among the most outstanding trainees I've ever had in almost two decades as well as a caring and sensitive person, and I've worked with some pretty awesome people.

Love
Laura

From: Laura
Sent: Wednesday, April 11, 2007 8:28 AM
To: Mel
Subject: Kindred spirits

Dear Mel,
Thanks for your beautiful letter. I see that we are kindred spirits.
I didn't know about your health problems—I am so sorry that you had to go through that! I am inspired by your

survival, but it doesn't surprise me about you. If you can make it through an aortic dissection, maybe I can handle a pinch of lymphoma!

I am writing a book about the experience of being a doctor and a patient. I'm thinking of calling it "Both Sides Now" (like the Judy Collins song).

I still look for justice in the universe, in spite of all evidence to the contrary. For some things I can't find the justice. Maybe that's where faith comes in. I didn't think I had much of that, but I'm finding more comfort in the prayer stuff than I would have believed possible.

I will send you updates. Thank you for agreeing to meet with Jung-min. I love her like a daughter.

Love
Laura

<hr>

From: Laura
Sent: Wednesday, April 11, 2007 8.45 PM
To: Mel
Subject: Backstory: David

Dear Mel,

I got an email back from the fellowship program director at your hospital. It looks like she is one of the good guys! I told Jung-min that she should look for you when she visits, and that you would look out for her. You will love her too.

You are right when you talk about how we meet at meetings and know so little about each other. Let me tell you more.

I met my husband, David, the summer before my freshman year in college. I was 16 (I had skipped a couple of years in school) and David was 19. He was my lab partner in Physics at Harvard Summer School. I was sitting in class on the first day in a pair of very short shorts (it was the seventies). David walked in: long black hair, moustache and beard, old beat-up sneakers, blue t- shirt, cozy flannel overshirt, and faded jeans, with a Dos Passos novel in his back pocket. He had a choice of sitting next to me or a woman with very large breasts named Liane who went to Wellesley. Luckily he picked me. I was especially lucky because I had originally signed up to study mime and juggling in Paris, Maine that summer, and switched to Physics at the last minute. Otherwise, I might have married a juggler!

After class, we went out for coffee together at a little café in the Harvard Science Center. He told me his name was David. I told him my name was Laura and that I had a brother named David (his age) and he said he had a sister named Laura (my age, living in Hollywood). When he revealed that his grandmother had a parakeet with the same name as my parakeet (Blue Boy), I knew that we were meant to be together. I found out quickly that he was a jazz enthusiast and was missing it terribly in Boston. He had brought two jazz mixed tapes and a small tape player, and listened to those tapes constantly. We shared a love of music; I'd previously listened primarily to classical music, but he introduced me to jazz.

A couple of nights after we met, I had to go get groceries in Harvard Square. David needed some stuff and asked me to pick it up and gave me his key to drop the stuff off in his room. I made a copy of his key. I didn't realize that this was a big deal, something that got discussed—I was just being practical. I figured I'm going to be spending time with this guy, so I need a key. I also got him one of those Hallmark cards that said, "Love is where you find it... I'll be here all day." And I wrote in: "...and for the rest of your life." Why he didn't run screaming in the other direction I can't imagine.

We were long distance for four years in college—he went to Dartmouth and I went to Harvard—and we had a commuter bus ticket from Boston to White River Junction, Vermont. He was a year ahead of me in school, so he graduated first. He went to medical school in New York, and I followed him to New York when I graduated college. We lived together for two years in medical school and then got married. I had basically asked him to marry me the summer we met; a mere six years later, he said yes. (But the company line is, he got down on bended knee and begged me to be his wife. That's our story and we're sticking to it.)

David and I have known each other 31 years out of the 47 I've been alive, and we celebrate our 25th wedding anniversary this June. He's a doctor specializing in Infectious Disease at Beth Israel in downtown New York, and does a lot of clinical work and research with AIDS patients. David is the most amazing husband and father. We go to jazz clubs together, and read books and hang out with the kids. He is my bird—we mated for life.

If I had to have cancer, I couldn't have picked a better partner to help me through it. Sometimes I think it's harder on the spouse than it is on the cancer patient. My mission is focused and defined (survival), while David has to pick up the pieces, emotionally support me and the kids, and deal with all the logistics of daily life. I tell the women faculty that one of the most important decisions they make is about a life partner. Life throws you a lot of curve balls, and if you're going to choose a partner, it should be someone who'll actually help. Unfortunately, by the time they're women faculty they've often made the choice already, and that ship has sailed. Sometimes I think the best thing we could do in the Women's Office is to find a bunch of suitable Significant Others for our women faculty, but I bet that's way beyond our budget.

Love
Laura

From: Laura
Sent: Thursday, April 12, 2007 8:47 PM
To: Mel
Subject: Backstory: Dad

Dear Mel,

Thanks for your email. I loved the story of how your parents met when your father was pumping gas in a gas station and your mother was in the car with her step-mother. I'm sorry that they each lost a parent at a young age. It's interesting that the lesson they taught you as a child was that everything you have could quickly be taken away from you. You asked about my parents, so I'll tell you.

My father, Robert Liberman, grew up in Chicago in the Depression. His dad died when he was six years old. He and his mom lived with relatives who argued all the time. My father was a peace-loving man who would walk 20 miles to avoid an argument. Being dependent on cantankerous relatives taught him the importance of being able to make your own living. "Be financially independent" was the take-home message of my childhood. My dad was a gifted pianist and had studied with Vladimir Horowitz's teacher. He could have been a concert pianist, but he hated to travel. More importantly, having grown up poor, he wanted a steady income.

The year my father graduated from high school, Sears/Roebuck gave a full tuition scholarship to the student who graduated first in his class from John Marshall High School, where my dad went. That person was my father. Being #2 would not have been good enough. That's how I learned to go for the top. He went to the University of Chicago (his home town) courtesy of Sears, joined the Army in World War II, and then attended Law School courtesy of the Army. When I went to college, it was a great source of pride to him that he could help pay for my education.

My dad was a law professor at Boston University. Law was an interesting career choice for a man who hated an argument. He practiced law only briefly. He mainly taught, and he was a wonderful teacher. He never pretended to know something he didn't—instead, he asked someone who knew, looked it up, or figured it out himself. I learned that lesson from him, and it's crucial, especially in medicine, where it can be life-threatening to pretend you know something you don't.

He used to take me out on Sunday mornings to breakfast at a Jewish deli in Boston called the B&D, and he taught me how to do algebra problems on the back of a paper napkin. John is two years older than Mary. In one year, John will be twice as old as Mary is now. How old are John and Mary? And I was always amazed that my father knew so many Johns and so many Marys.

My father met my mother on a blind date when she was in law school and he was a practicing lawyer. A friend asked him if he wanted to meet a cute blonde or a big Israeli. He chose the big Israeli, Judith (now Judith Weinshall Liberman)—that's my mom. She's tall, about 5'10"; he was 5'7". She got the best grades in the class and worked the hardest. In a Master of Laws program they took after they got married, my mom studied like crazy; my dad just skimmed her notes the night before the exam.

She got the highest score and he got the next highest—a hair lower, but with much less work. She laughs when she tells the story. I was a student in my mom's tradition of relentless workaholism, while my husband was a more inspired and laid back student like my dad. My mom gave up law to be an artist, while my dad became a law professor.

Having pulled himself up from poverty, my father knew the value of hard work. He used to quote Thomas Edison, who said, "Genius is 1% inspiration and 99% perspiration." We used to play the card game, "Hearts." Usually, in Hearts, every heart you win counts one point against you, and the Queen of Spades counts 13 points against you. However, winning all of the hearts and the Queen of Spades is a landslide victory called "shooting the moon." My dad always tried to shoot the moon, and usually succeeded. He taught me to try even when the outcome was uncertain. Again, he quoted Edison: when Edison's initial attempts to invent the light bulb did not yield the results he hoped, he said, "I have not failed. I've just found 10,000 ways that don't work."

When I was in high school, Stanford was my top choice for college. I looked at the map of the country and saw that Palo Alto, California was about as far as you could go in the United States from Newton, Massachusetts, and figured that's what I had to do to be independent. Luckily I was rejected. Maybe they thought I was too young at 16. But I picked up the broken pieces of my life and went to Harvard. Proximity to my family turned out to be a wonderful thing. My father had a heart attack the summer after my freshman year in college and then multiple strokes after that, and spent much of the next few years in and out of the hospital. Because I was in school so close to home, I was able to spend precious time with him.

While I was growing up, my father loved to play the piano. I remember falling asleep at night listening to him playing Chopin Nocturnes (how many girls are lucky enough to get that kind of lullaby?). Encouraged by my father, I started playing the piano when I was six. When I was ten and again when I was twelve, I was the guest piano soloist with the Boston Symphony Orchestra. We had two pianos at home, a small upright and a big grand piano, both in our living room. We played piano duets together, for fun and in concerts. My favorite was the Schubert Fantastia in F Minor, where the voices of the two pianos echo and complement each other like two inseparable friends.

My father loved to read and analyze literature. He was a terrific writer and published short stories. A gentle soul, he wrote surprisingly dark stories, some of which reflected memories of German concentration camps that he had seen in World War II. He loved to read books about the process of writing, like The Technique of the Novel by Thomas Uzzell. I got my love of reading and writing from him, and have passed it on to Nate and Emma. He would have loved to write a novel, but he got stuck in the outline phase. Years of outlines, covering one yellow legal pad after another with his exuberant handwriting in black ink.

I remember speaking to him one night right after he had the stroke that robbed him of his ability to play the piano. I have never heard a voice so broken by loss. He told me that he was sorry I had been born, because he did not want me to get hurt someday as he had been hurt. He said, "Why couldn't I have brought someone into the world who is heartless, cruel, cold, and unfeeling? The world is no place for sensitive people."

When he was in the hospital, he had slurred speech from the stroke, but his mind was lucid. I remember how some of the doctors and nurses treated him like he was stupid because he couldn't enunciate his words clearly. I couldn't believe what a difference it made to his outlook and self-esteem whether he was treated with respect and compassion or with the assumption that he was an idiot.

My father had always wanted me to be a doctor. When I was six years old and playing the piano, people would ask my father, "What does Laura want to be?" And he said, "She wants to be a concert pianist, but medicine will be her back-up profession." I remember thinking, "I never said that. That must be what *he* wants." When my father got sick during my college years, I gave up my physics major (which I had particularly enjoyed because I was the only girl in the class) and decided to be a doctor. I figured that's what he wanted, and I loved him so much that I wanted it too. Maybe I could keep people from suffering the way he suffered.

My father taught me what it takes to master something. He used to practice the piano for hours daily. He used to say, "If I don't practice one day, I know it; if I don't practice two days, my friends know it; if I don't practice three days, the audience knows it." After the first stroke, he was tireless at doing his rehabilitation exercises. He spent hours relearning activities like putting on socks, tying his shoes, and walking. He never got impatient or frustrated; if he didn't succeed, he would simply do it again. Once I went to rehab with him, and I remember how he asked the therapist to give him more exercises. "I'm very good at practicing," he told her. He was right.

My father died right after I began my radiology residency in New York. He had spent much of the last few years of his life terrified of becoming a vegetable from another stroke. As it turned out, he worried for nothing—he died of a massive heart attack in the middle of a chess game, and he was a knight and a pawn ahead at the time. If my father had only known that would be his exit strategy, the last few years of his life would have been so much better! He would have particularly enjoyed that at the moment of his death during the chess game, he was winning.

He wanted to be cremated and have his ashes scattered in the ocean. On the morning of his funeral, I couldn't believe that the sun was shining as if nothing had happened. We rented a boat in Maine, and released his ashes with Beethoven's 7th Symphony, 2nd movement (Allegro) playing. I chose that music because it combines major and minor keys, expressing how life is full of both sorrow and joy: it's sad that he died, but it's even more glorious that he lived. The score starts with a simple base line, and then progressively adds more and more instruments until there is a groundswell of unbelievably beautiful music, analogous to starting at birth, finding more complexity and joy at each level of life, and finally earning the ascent into heaven.

During the funeral, I was comforted by the fact that my father had met and liked David, and that he got to attend our wedding three years before he died. However, I was seized by the thought that now my kids (who were not even a twinkle in my eye at that point!) would never get to meet my father. It was an odd thought. Until then I hadn't been certain about having children, but when I lost my father, I realized that having kids was no longer a question of whether, only when. I wish I could talk to my father again, even just for five minutes, and I wish he could meet Nate and Emma. Talk about a sense of humor. He had it all.

That's my story. Maybe that's how I'll tell it in the book. The book may end up being emails that I write and receive during this journey. If it's OK with you, I may include the picture you sent me of the seed becoming a plant that grew right through the roof of your hot tub. That was a beautiful picture and a beautiful story. I hope to be strong like the seed, and to break through hot tub covers in a single bound.

Love
Laura

From: Laura
Sent: Friday, April 13, 2007 5:36 AM
To: Mark
Subject: Pain: ideas

Hi Mark. I want to touch base with you in your capacity as a neurosurgeon about something important. I've had four Omaya taps for intrathecal chemo so far, so I speak from some experience. My lymphoma doc is a wonderful doctor and a terrific human being. The procedure itself, however, is painful.

Sometimes, as doctors, we feel that the most important aspect of treatment is killing the cancer, and if that means you feel a little pain, you should "suck it up." I agree that if killing the cancer requires pain, suck it up. But if the cancer can be cured in a way that is painful or less painful but equally effective, the less painful method is the clear choice.

There is a feeling (of which I have also been guilty, when I got to play doctor) that focusing on the pain distracts from the major mission of curing the cancer. That's wrong. Even if the physician who has primary responsibility for killing the cancer doesn't want to be "distracted" by thinking about pain, we should make it a priority that someone on the team is focused on pain relief. We should not tolerate errors in pain management any more than we would tolerate giving the wrong dose of chemo, or treating with an improper antibiotic, or performing surgery on the wrong side of the body.

I have specific suggestions for pain prevention when putting a needle into an Omaya. For the past few decades in

Breast Imaging, we've been doing pre-operative needle localization procedures, in which we place a wire in a woman's breast pre-operatively to guide the surgeon towards a breast lesion that can't be felt. Before the loc, we spray the area of the breast with a spray called "Gebauer's Ethyl Chloride Medium Stream Spray," which is considered a "topical anesthetic skin refrigerant" and works instantly. Another good local anesthetic is Emla cream. It can be applied over the area to be accessed (eg the Omaya or Mediport), but unlike the spray, the Emla cream requires half an hour to work.

Since you put the Omayas in during neurosurgery, is there a way you can convey in the post-op instructions the recommendation for numbing prior to putting a needle into the Omaya to remove fluid or give chemo? You can even suggest the Ethyl Chloride spray and the Emla cream. Either the treating oncologist could give the patient the necessary prescriptions, or we can make sure that the meds are available in all the chemo suites so that they can be used to increase patient comfort for all needling procedures. The spray or Emla cream could also be used prior to other needling procedures elsewhere in the body, like accessing Mediports. After the anesthesia, the area can be prepped with sterile technique, so it shouldn't increase the chance of infection.

Another thing. I learned through personal experience that the likelihood of vomiting is directly related to the speed of intrathecal injection. Sam, my neurologist, confirmed that if it's injected too quickly, once it hits the 4th ventricle it tickles the vomiting center and you puke. If we're rewriting the post-Omaya instructions, can we include the recommendation to inject slowly, and maybe even give a guideline as to the maximum suggested injection rate? Most intrathecal chemo patients probably believe that vomiting just goes with the territory, and would not think to ask the physician to slow down. We need to write it into the guidelines to make it happen.

I'd appreciate your thoughts. I am no wimp and if pain is necessary to cure my lymphoma, I'll endure it. But if we can make it less painful or even painless, we should go for it. Even a small amount of pain per procedure over a long course of treatment adds up, and gives those individuals with cancer yet another thing to dread. It is our mission not only to cure cancer but also to relieve suffering. We can be the best at both. Let's do it. Then I will know that my lymphoma is for a good reason, and I will find the justice in the universe that I perpetually seek.

Best wishes
And in a spirit of making things better (always)
Laura

Chapter 9
Blurry Vision

Get your priorities straight.

From: Laura
Sent: Friday, April 13, 2007 8:26 PM
To: Sam
Subject: Blurry vision: questions

Hi Sam. Question for you about my eyes—I have worsening blurry vision the last few days, which makes it difficult to read (but doesn't stop me from sending an email!).

I've been near-sighted requiring glasses since I was six years old. I started to have trouble reading several months ago, and now have "progressives," which I gather are the new "bifocals." When I began having the neuro symptoms that led to the eventual diagnosis of lymphoma, I saw Jack of Ophthalmology here, who saw a few cells in my eyes that were suspicious for lymphoma (apparently that's reasonably frequent if you have lymphoma in the CSF). .

Now I've finished four intrathecal methotrexates, two IV R-CHOPS, and one high-dose IV methotrexate, with the most recent intrathecal methotrexate and IV R-CHOP being this past Tuesday 4/10 (which I tolerated fine). In the past several days I've noticed a worsening of blurry vision, which makes it difficult to read. Could this be related to the steroids (I'm on day three of five days of oral prednisone through Sunday 4/15)? If it is due to the prednisone, is the blurry vision likely to get better when I'm off prednisone? I'm especially concerned because my eyes are key in radiology, especially breast imaging—you have to be sharp if you're going to pick up the tiny microcalcifications that may be the only sign of an early breast cancer. Alternatively, could the visual blurring be due to worsening lymphoma of the eyes, especially in light of the abnormal cells in my eyes before I began treatment?

Should I have labs checked (and if so, which labs and when, and can you put in and release the orders)? My next scheduled appointment with my oncologist is on Thursday 4/19 at noon, when I am scheduled to get more intrathecal chemo. Should I make another appointment with Jack, see my outside eye doctor to get my prescription checked, or just wait until Thursday and see my oncologist then? Thanks for your advice!

Laura

From: Laura
Sent: Saturday, April 14, 2007 4:32 AM
To: Jennifer
Subject: Saturday

Hi Jen. We had a great day yesterday. In the morning, David rented a car to take Emma and me to a parent-teacher conference at Emma's school. I wore a hat called the Gordon, a straw fedora in a muted pink with flip brim and silk gray trim.

I was so proud of Emma at the conference. Going from elementary school to high school is a big transition, even without having a sick mom, and she's been handling it beautifully. Emma came to the conference with us, and became a little shy when her advisor read all the fabulous comments from her teachers. Afterwards, Emma went to class. David dropped me off at the hospital and went to work.

110

The main event on my calendar at work today was a meeting about "the MSK Nanny Resource," an internal list-serve we're creating to address the issue of child care for employees. We brainstormed this idea with Amy and Nancy, my colleagues in Work/Life, after we collaborated on a seminar called "How to Find a Nanny." On the Nanny Resource, employees can post if they want to hire or share a nanny, or if they have a great nanny they no longer need. We met with the information technology guy, Kevin, who was helpful. We left with a list of things to do, all doable. I think it will happen!

Every month we put a new "Quote of the Month" on the Women Faculty Affairs website. This month we're posting a poem by Emily Dickinson. I think you'll like it.

Hope is the thing with feathers by Emily Dickinson

Hope is the thing with feathers
That perches in the soul,
And sings the tune without the words,
And never stops at all,

 And sweetest in the gale is heard;
And sore must be the storm
That could abash the little bird
That kept so many warm.

I've heard it in the chillest land
And on the strangest sea;
Yet, never, in extremity,
It asked a crumb of me.

Love
Laura

From: Laura
Sent: Sunday, April 15, 2007 7:29 PM
To: Jennifer
Subject: Bird by Bird

Hi Jen. Today I spent most of the day rereading one of my favorite books, Anne Lamott's *Bird by Bird*. Although the book is ostensibly about writing, it might just as well be about dealing with cancer. The title story is derived from an incident in which the author's big brother, as a kid, was assigned to write an essay about the birds of North America. He found the task overwhelming. When his father asked him what the problem was, Lamott's brother said that there were a lot of birds in North America. His father looked at him reassuringly and said, "Bird by bird, buddy. Just take it bird by bird."

The story reminds me of advice Maureen gave me shortly after I was diagnosed, when I was considering declining treatment. She told me I don't have to agree to the whole deal; I could just agree to start, and then take it one day at a time. The advice was comforting. This approach let me maintain the illusion of control ("it's no illusion; you ARE in control," Maureen would say). It also broke up the impossible task of six months of chemo into a series of manageable tasks, dealing with each individual day. I would do it bird by bird.

Love
Laura

From: Laura
Sent: Monday, April 16, 2007 4:56 AM
To: Jennifer
Subject: Broadway

Hi Jen. Q and I went to see the Eugene O'Neill play "Moon for the Misbegotten" starring Kevin Spacey on Broadway yesterday, and it was fabulous. I decided to wear a hat that didn't go up too high on my head, so I wouldn't block the view of the person sitting behind me. I chose the Reese paisley, which has a fabric slouch crown with a split cuff brim and a "self trim," which means part of the same fabric as the hat serves as the trim. The fabric is a subtle silver, beige, and black paisley pattern, with a small sewn silk flower at the side.

The play was great, but it desperately needed editing. If I were an English professor, I would assign my students to cut an hour off of it—the run time was almost 3 hours. It took me two nausea pills at $40/pill (that Zofran is worth its weight in gold) to get through the play. If the play had been an hour shorter, I could have done it in one nausea pill. Do you think the estate of Eugene O'Neill would listen to reason? They owe me 40 bucks.

The hardest part of the outing was afterwards, when Q and I went to get a cab. It was rainy and the streets were slippery. As I was getting into the cab I slipped and almost fell, and then hit my head (the part with the Omaya) against the cab. I started to cry. Q helped me up and pulled me into the cab and gave me a hug, which I desperately needed. I try to be brave and optimistic about all this, but the bottom line is that cancer makes you feel vulnerable, and I used to feel invincible.

I don't remember if I told you—I started having severe visual blurring, which is bothersome, because reading and writing are integral in my life right now. The blurring began around the time I started my latest course of prednisone. Sam, my neurologist, said that visual blurring is common on prednisone. Apparently the symptoms can be triggered by either raising or lowering the steroid dose but usually disappear after steroids are stopped. Steroids can also cause cataracts or glaucoma. These possible side effects are not good news, but all of them are better than having the visual blurring represent worsening lymphoma in my eyes. Yesterday I took my last dose of prednisone for the month, so hopefully the symptoms will improve. I'm still going to see the eye doctor to make sure.

My father is on my mind a lot these days. I'm listening to piano music that he played, like Schumann's Kreisleriana; he especially liked part 1, for which the tempo marking is "agitatissimo," or very agitated. The piece is fiendishly difficult, requiring a massive reach for both hands. My father used to tell me how Schumann injured his right hand, possibly as the result of a mechanical device he used to increase the strength, independence, and span of his fingers. Apparently Schumann became psychologically unstable, and spent the last two years of his life in a mental institution. Schumann's wife, Clara, an excellent pianist who was the daughter of Schumann's boyhood piano teacher, was the one who held it together in their family. Any frustration my father ever felt was released in the Olympic-level workout of the Kreisleriana.

My father loved to play Beethoven sonatas, especially the ones that were the most technically challenging. I've been listening to one of his favorites, Beethoven's "Appassionata" Sonata #23 Op. 57. I remember him playing the third movement, with a tempo marking "allegro ma non troppo" (fast but not too fast). As I watched his fingers fly across the keys, I doubted that it was possible to play it any faster. My dad used to tell me that Beethoven started to lose his hearing in his twenties and was completely deaf by age 50. It struck me as ironic that a man who was so passionate about composing music lost his hearing. I thought about Beethoven going deaf when my father lost his manual dexterity and his piano playing after a stroke.

I've been listening to Mozart sonatas that my father and I played together. One of my father's favorite books was a biography of Mozart by Marcia Davenport. My father loved to tell me stories about Wolfgang Amadeus Mozart: when Mozart was three, he watched his older sister Nannerl play the piano; when he was four, his father Leopold started to give him piano lesions; he began composing at age five; and he spent his subsequent childhood traveling with Leopold all over Europe, performing as a child prodigy. My dad always said that Mozart wrote more than 600 priceless compositions, but died "a poor churchmouse" at age 35. I knew that if my dad had been Wolfgang's father, he would have encouraged him to find a better paying job.

One of the first pieces my father and I played together was the Mozart Sonata for 1 piano, 4 hands, in D Major, KV 381/123a. I used to laugh when our hands got tangled up as one of us reached over the other for a trill or arpeggio outside of our own "turf." As I got older, we each wanted to have an entire keyboard to ourselves, so we preferred music for two pianos, like the Mozart D Major Piano Sonata, K. 448. To this day, D Major still feels to me like a joyful key of innocence and youth. Listening to the music my dad played, and especially to the music we played together, makes me feel like he's up there looking out for me.

Love
Laura

From: Laura
Sent: Monday, April 16, 2007 5:22 PM
To: Jennifer
Subject: Emily Dickinson

Hi Jen. Today at work I wore a hat called the Roz, a two-piece cloche in black and brown with a curved pheasant feather rising up from the side. On the way to a meeting, I was in the elevator with an elderly couple. The wife was looking at me and speaking to her husband in Italian. I smiled at her and said, "You're talking about my hat, aren't you?" And she said to me in a thick Italian accent, "Yes. I love your hat!" When I'm wearing these hats, I never worry about making conversation.

I found a poem that captures my feelings about how I want to use my experience with pain to help others:

- -

If I can stop one heart from breaking by Emily Dickinson

If I can stop one heart from breaking
I shall not live in vain;
If I can ease one life the aching
Or cool one pain,
Or help one fainting robin
Unto his nest again,
I shall not live in vain.

- -

Love
Laura

From: PWFA/President's Office
Sent: Monday, April 16, 2007 12:48 PM
To: All Women Faculty
Subject: Athena Tuesday 4/24, 5 pm

To Women Faculty:
    Please come to the next ATHENA, our informal women faculty group, on Tues 4/24 5-7 pm, Faculty Club. Come for a few minutes or stay longer. I hope you'll join us!

Best wishes
Laura

Laura Liberman, M.D.
Director, Program for Women Faculty Affairs

From: Laura
Sent: Monday, April 16, 2007 7:58 PM
To: Jimmie
Subject: Your amazing book!

    Hi Jimmie. Thank you for sending me your amazing, wonderful, awesome, incredible book, *The Human Side of Cancer*, which is exactly what I need to read right now! I feel like you wrote it for me. After I finish reading it, can we talk? You are a fantastic writer!
    Also, thanks for sending me the Stephen Gould book, *Full House: The Spread of Excellence from Plato to Darwin*. I especially liked the chapter called "Case One, A Personal Story:

Where any measure of a central tendency acts as a harmful abstraction, and variation stands out as the only meaningful reality." Basically, Gould seems to be saying that even if the median survival of your cancer is 50% at one year, that means half of the people with that cancer live less than one year, but half live more—and some people may live ten, twenty, thirty years or longer. This news is particularly good for people like me, who are told that their illness has a lousy median survival. When I saw Figure 7 on page 55, I imagined myself way on the right, at the highest end of the survival bell curve, waving and smiling.

Your book and Gould's should be recommended for every cancer patient.

Best wishes
Laura

From: Laura
Sent: Tuesday, April 17, 2007 2:13 AM
To: Jennifer
Subject: Nate's college forms

Hi Jen. Nate is working on his college applications. We started to talk about colleges last summer (the summer before his junior year) when we were on vacation in Hilton Head, South Carolina. Nate and I biked over to the only tiny book store in town and bought the one copy of the *Fiske Guide to Colleges*. I suggested that Nate make an Excel spread sheet listing the colleges he was considering and their characteristics, to organize his thinking. It was an opportunity for me to teach

Nate an important lesson: many of life's problems can be solved, or at least helped, by a good Excel spreadsheet.

Today Nate started to work on the nitty gritty of applying to college. The process at Nate's school is very organized. They have all these forms and questionnaires for the students to fill out in preparation for a meeting with the college counselor. Students have to express their interests, talk about the subjects they enjoy, and describe what their extracurricular activities have been. The parents have to fill out forms too. Nate's interests have been non-traditional, centering on teaching and community service.

Nate's first exposure to working with kids was when he was in fifth grade, and his elementary school partnered each fifth grader to a first grader in their "buddy class." The summer after eighth grade, Nate was a camp counselor for a group of 5-year-olds. I know the students adored him because one summer day a 5-year-old girl in his group recognized him as we were walking down the block and ran up to him to give him a hug. She hugged his knees, because they were as high as she could reach. The girl's mom, who recognized Nate, said to her daughter, "Do you know who that is?" And the girl said, "That's Nate, my counselor!" as if he were a rock star.

When Nate went to high school, he started tutoring third-graders in a bilingual Spanish/English public school on the West Side. One student drew a crayon picture of Nate as a superhero, complete with uniform, sword, and shield; it's still hanging on Nate's wall. Nate told us about a girl in the class who failed a math test. On one question in which she was asked to draw a triangle with vertices C, A, T, she had drawn a cat, not a triangle. Instead of berating her, Nate commented on the realism of her drawing, and asked, do you have a cat? What's the cat's name? What kind of cat is it? The girl was so engaged that when he started to explain the math to her, she listened.

During the summer after he finished ninth grade, Nate volunteered at a neighborhood soup kitchen that gave groceries to individuals and families in need. I thought it was just a summer gig, but he kept it up weekly throughout high school. He rose through the ranks and eventually ran the line for distributing food to the elderly and disabled. I was proud of his dedication. During the subsequent summer and school year, he also volunteered to teach in a program to help low-income New York City elementary school kids prepare to apply to challenging public or private high schools. A student of Nate's became one of the first three students in the program to get admitted to a New York Independent School. Nate described these experiences in his college essay.

I like the way Nate writes: get your thoughts down on paper first and edit later. That's a method Anne Lamott suggests in the chapter "Shitty First Drafts" in her book, *Bird by Bird*. I think getting any thoughts down on paper and then cleaning it up is a great strategy because it takes an impossible task (taking the blank page and filling it with a beautiful story) and breaks it into two smaller, easier tasks (writing the "shitty first draft," and then editing work you've already written).

It wasn't only Nate writing today—David and I had to fill out parent college forms. In addition to the name, rank, and serial number stuff, they asked us to specifically name where we would like him to apply to college. We wrote down that we wanted him to go where he wants to go, so he can be happy. I don't understand pressuring your kids to go to the same school you did. Your kids are not you; they have their own tastes, interests, and abilities, and need to find schools that are right for them.

The college application process with Nate has taught me that parenting a teenager is like getting a bird to eat out of your hand. You love the bird; you want to feed the bird; you have

120

only the bird's best interests at heart; you would never, ever hurt the bird. But if you make big sudden movements, the bird will fly away. You have to be casual. You stroll over, toss out a few seeds, and step back, like you don't even notice. Maybe he won't come at first. But then each day you put out a few more seeds and step back. Eventually he may come, and maybe at some point (if you're very lucky!) he'll take a seed before he bolts and then another and another and finally one day you'll feel the tickle of his beak in your hand before he flies away.

Love
Laura

From: Laura
Sent: Tuesday, April 17, 2007 9:40 AM
To: Maureen
Subject: Athena

Hi Maureen. Question for you. There is an Athena gathering on Tues 4/24 from 5-7 pm in the Faculty Club. I am getting admitted for chemo that day. Can you lead this Athena? There are a few announcements to make, and basically I want someone to be there to make people feel welcome. Would this be OK?

Do you want to pop by here this morning (I'm in the women's office) and catch up for a few? I'm going to the Junior Faculty Council meeting at noon.

I'm doing OK. Intrathecal chemo Thursday, another admission Tuesday. Have finished seven of 18 doses of chemo—only 11 left. After the next admission is done, I'll have finished nine of 18 chemos—the halfway mark.

Love
Laura

From: Laura
Sent: Thursday, April 19, 2007 2:08 AM
To: Jennifer
Subject: Seminar

Hi Jen. I loved what you said about how nobody calls you Jenny. It's like with Nate. When he was born, David and I named him Nathaniel, and figured we would call him by that name. But from the moment of his birth, he's been such a thorough and complete Nate. We have a video of bringing him home from the hospital right after he was born. We carried him over the threshold and said, "Welcome home, Nathaniel." I don't think we've called him Nathaniel since. I remember once when he was three, a friend's mom called him "Nathaniel." Nate said, "Don't call me Nathaniel. My name is Nate!" I was shocked that my three-year-old was so certain of his own identity. On rare occasions, some people call him Nathaniel, but he's mostly Nate to those of us who know him best.

I went to a fabulous career development seminar today. I wore a hat called the Tracy, which had a beige straw cloth square crown with a large down brim and muted green hand rolled roses. The seminar was jointly run by Cornell, Columbia, Sinai, Einstein, and NYU. Sometimes these seminars get a little whiney, but this one had the best speakers, and there were terrific people to meet.

A woman who is Director of Diversity at Columbia University spoke about diversity in the workplace, and was absolutely spectacular! She talked about how people (women and men) are looking for balance in their lives now, and it's no longer acceptable for many of them to work 24/7. I know this to be true. I also think we pay the consequences for our overwork. Relentless stress takes its toll on our psyches, bodies, spirits, and families.

We have to figure out a way to let people work but also let their work lives fit with the rest of their lives. Even if the goal is simply to get as much work as possible out of a person, it is better strategy to allow them to try to make the pieces fit. Life is a marathon, not a sprint. If you give all your steam on the first leg of the relay you'll have nothing left for the finale. I know that this is true, but how do we make it a reality when we are all such Type A personalities, want nothing short of perfection, and work in a cancer hospital where the stakes are high and mistakes can have lethal consequences?

Another amazing speaker at the conference was named Catherine J. Morrison, J.D. She gave two terrific sessions, a general lecture on negotiation and a seminar on conflict resolution. I especially liked her Frank Zappa quote: "Reality is an optional experience!" I'm going to follow up with her and see if she can give a session for our women faculty.

At the seminar, a female junior faculty member who took a grantwriting course sponsored by Women Faculty Affairs just found out that she was awarded her grant from the National Institutes of Health! Isn't that fantastic, wonderful news? This Women Faculty Affairs job is great—I get to play Point Guard. I feel like Teresa Weatherspoon of the New York Liberty in the WNBA: I get the ball to the Center, and she gets it into the net.

The seminar was held at Columbia University, which is gorgeous—a beautiful college campus right in the middle of New York City. After the seminar, I went to the college bookstore and bought a CD of classic Beatles tunes to put on my iPod. I'm still listening to a lot of music these days, especially when I'm in the hospital or getting chemo.

The only bad thing about today is that my vision is still blurry. It's hard to see the traffic signs across the street. I never realized how scary it is to go out in the world unable to see.

Love
Laura

Chapter 10
Good News, Bad News

It's OK to cry, but do so ≤20 minutes/day.

From: Laura
Sent: Thursday, April 19, 2007 9:28 PM
To: Jennifer
Subject: Good news/bad news

Hi Jen. I got good news and bad news today. The good news is that my visual blurring is probably due to prednisone. The bad news is that my cerebrospinal fluid (CSF) won't clear—it still has atypical lymphocytes. If these lymphocytes are lymphoma, and they can't get rid of them, I probably won't survive.

Now I'm going to go cry (less than 20 minutes), and then I'll sit at the lap top and write and feel better. There's more to tell but I'm exhausted. I'll write later.

Love
Laura

From: Laura
Sent: Friday, April 20, 2007 1:28 AM
To: Jennifer
Subject: Highs and lows

Dearest Jen,

OK, I'm here to fill in the details about yesterday, which was the toughest day I've had yet. Emotional highs and lows. I'm exhausted thinking about it and it hurts to tell it, but it's going in the book, so I better go ahead.

It started with an appointment with the ophthalmologist. I told you I've been having blurry vision for about a week now, since I got the last dose of R-CHOP. My near vision is OK, but my distance vision is screwed up. When I went to the play on Sunday, Kevin Spacey was a fuzzy blur moving across the stage. Having blurry vision in the middle of Manhattan is scary. But the most terrifying thing about the blurry vision was thinking about what it could mean. The blurry vision may be from the prednisone, which changes the curvature of the lens of the eye (the lens gets swollen and puffy like everything else on steroids) or it could be from worsening lymphoma in the eyes.

I saw Jack, the ophthalmic oncology guy recommended by my neurologist. Jack is a man of few words, tall and thin, a little older than me, personable, and extremely knowledgeable. He tested both eyes, took measurements for a new prescription, and said that my blurry vision is because of the steroids. Decline in vision is apparently very common, particularly at the beginning of R-CHOP treatment, and usually stabilizes at a certain point. He saw no abnormal cells in my eyes, so it's NOT worsening ocular lymphoma. He wants me to come back on Monday so that he can recheck my vision, and if Monday's prescription is stable from yesterday's, he wants me to get new glasses.

I was thrilled about the good news. The ability to see (which lets me read and write) is essential for me. If I have to choose between seeing and hearing, I'd pick seeing, although I hope I won't have to make that particular choice.

I had another intrathecal chemotherapy. I was starving and brought my lunch (a fresh salad that I made in the cafeteria) with me to eat while I was waiting for chemo. When Phil came in to tap the Omaya and I was eating a salad, he said, "You're eating before the chemo?" I told him that I was hungry, and that I also wanted him to see what I was having for lunch, because I knew he would not want to make me throw up and see it a second time. I told Phil that I had learned that if I throw up, it's because he's injecting too fast. I said that if that happens, I'm going to aim directly for his soft brown leather imported Italian shoes, and that when I take aim, I do not miss. Guess what? Phil injected slowly, and I didn't puke! Afterwards, I sat with Cindy and she held pressure on my head (which bled awhile) until I felt OK.

After we finished the intrathecal chemo, I had a serious discussion with Phil about the fact that my CSF (the cerebrospinal fluid surrounding the brain and spinal cord) has not cleared. Yesterday was my fifth dose of intrathecal methotrexate. Before each injection of intrathecal methotrexate, they take out some fluid (called "tapping the Omaya") and send it to the lab so they can analyze the cells under the microscope. We had originally planned six doses of intrathecal chemo, and Phil had thought that the CSF would clear after the first dose or two. Unfortunately, my Omaya taps still show atypical lymphocytes. Phil's sending the fluid from yesterday's tap for fancy tests (including something called "flow cytometry") to find out for sure whether these cells are lymphoma, but he suspects that they are. I should get those results on Monday.

If the flow cytometry is negative (meaning no lymphoma cells from the Omaya), then after my third cycle of chemo is done, they're going to do a lumbar puncture (LP, or spinal tap). I asked Phil why we need the LP if he's tapping the Omaya, and he said that the CSF around the brain (which is what you get in an Omaya tap) and the CSF around the spinal cord (which you get by doing an LP) mix with each other but sometimes the mixing is incomplete, and what you find in one might be different than what you find in the other. We'll need to send the fluid from the LP for flow cytometry also, so that we can thoroughly analyze all of the CSF for the presence of lymphoma.

Phil is thinking about changing me to even stronger intrathecal chemo. I'm worried. The intrathecal methotrexate I'm on now is tough to take, and I'm concerned that if they hit me with more aggressive intrathecal chemo for worsening lymphoma, either the stronger chemo or the lymphoma or both will kill me. I'm trying to stay positive and I'm still hoping to blow this cancer thing out of the water, but I'm also terrified of dying.

After my appointment, Cindy took me home in a cab. On the way home, she said she was going to be in the city on Saturday, and asked if I wanted to meet at St. Patrick's cathedral so we could light candles. It sounded like a comforting thing to do, so I said yes, and we made plans to meet there at 4 pm on Saturday.

When I got home, I was upset about two things. First, there is a chronic leak in our master bathroom, which has been overgrown with fungus for months. It could probably kill a healthy person, but with my low white blood cell count it is a death zone. Second, we have a beautiful terrace on which we planted flowers and trees a few years ago. For the past two summers, they've been doing construction on the terrace. They killed the plants, broke the glass window panes, moved away our table to make room for their equipment, and rendered the space unusable. Now that I'm sick, I want to sit out there when the weather is warm enough and bring my lap top and write.

David has spoken multiple times to the new super about these problems (the old super was a crook who took bribes and got fired). The new super keeps saying that he will take care of

these things, but it hasn't happened yet. So today I had enough.
I intercommed the front desk and told them to send me the
super, that I had to speak to him personally. Nate and Carmen
were here. I told them to get ready for a scene.

Jesus, the new super, came. He is a quiet man in his 40's,
with a Spanish accent, medium build, and dark hair. I greeted
him with no hat, bald. I told him that I have cancer, that I'm
getting chemotherapy, and that there is a good chance that I'll
be dead within a year. I told him that I need him to get the
terrace finished so that I can sit out there. I showed him every
item on the terrace that needs to be fixed. Then I asked him to
go into our disgusting fungemic bathroom and told him that the
doctors said that this could kill me if it is not corrected
immediately. I told him that if I died because of the fungus in
the bathroom, he was responsible for my children losing their
mother. I screamed, I cried, and I begged him in the name of
God to help me.

By the time I was finished, poor Jesus was a shaking
shell of a human being. This quiet God-fearing gentleman had a
hysterical bald woman on his hands. I must have lit a fire under
him. He made a bunch of calls; he promised he would take care
of it; he gave me a hug and kissed my hand; and he said he goes
to church every day and will pray for me. He gave me his cell
phone number and told me I could call him any time of the day
or night. And then he left, but he must have been upset, because
he left his wallet in our apartment and had to come back to get it.

After the scene with Jesus, Emma came home. I had to
have a heart to heart talk with Emma about a bunch of things.
I've been showering in her bathroom in the mornings because
I've been afraid to go in the death zone of our master bathroom.
Sometimes the sound of my showering wakes her up. This
morning I couldn't find the hat I wanted to wear, and I looked in
her room, and I kept knocking on her door to come in, which

interrupted her sleep. And she hadn't slept well the night before. I knew she was irritated, but my kids don't want to be mad at me these days because I'm sick. I apologized for interrupting Emma's privacy to look for the hat. I told her I won't leave my hats in her room anymore. Together, we made a plan for when I can use her shower without disturbing her. I told her that it's OK for her to be upset, and that I was glad we could talk about what's been going on.

David came home. Jesus had called him, and David wanted to know what had happened. I explained the scene, after which David came up with all sorts of reasons why the plan of fixing the bathroom couldn't work. The Super had asked Carmen to clean out the bathroom, and Carmen started saying that she would do it in the morning. And then I lost it. David, Carmen, Emma, and I were in the family room, and Nate was in the living room at the table, working with his SAT II tutor. I started to scream.

I screamed that I needed them to do what I asked exactly the way I wanted. When Carmen asked me why I was getting so upset, I screamed "BECAUSE I'M SCARED I'M GOING TO DIE! IS THAT SO HARD TO UNDERSTAND?" I was told today that the CSF is not clearing, and I know that if the CSF doesn't clear, I won't live. I'm making the best effort I can to beat this thing, but ultimately whether I survive is beyond my control. Although there is a lot about which I can't call the shots, I'd like to control the few things I can. I want to sit on the terrace. I want a bathroom that is free of fungus. I want the people I love to help make that happen, and not tell me a thousand reasons why they can't. I hadn't even realized that was what made me so upset, and once I did and told them, they understood.

Poor Nate. He overheard my scream about "I'M SCARED I'M GOING TO DIE" in the living room with his tutor. Apparently he looked up sweetly at her and said in a calm voice, "I think we're done." She initially thought the screaming was from the neighbors, but apparently I screamed again, and then she realized, "The call is coming from inside the house." Nate is so funny when he tells the story.

I'm not scared of dying for me; I don't want to leave David and Nate and Emma. They deserve more.

Love
Laura

Chapter 11
Test Results

Ask people to pray for you. Get in shape. Go iPod.

From: Laura
Sent: Friday, Apr 20, 2007 2:17 AM
To: Phil
Subject: Treatment thoughts and questions

Hi Phil. Question: will I be getting intrathecal chemo when I see you at 9:45 am this Tuesday, prior to my admission that day? And do I come straight to you first for the appointment, and then go to the Admitting Office afterwards?

Don't worry about the ridiculously early time on the email. My sleep schedule is odd, but I'm getting enough sleep. I usually take my evening pharmacy of medicines around 8-9, sleep about four or five hours, wake up and write for a couple of hours, and then go to sleep until somewhere between 4 and 6 am. So I get about 6 hours of sleep a night (I have never been a good sleeper). The prednisone may contribute but I have a similar pattern off steroids.

I keep thinking about our last visit. I had so wanted the CSF cytology to clear and I'm concerned that it may not be clearing. If you need to switch to a bigger intrathecal gun, I will do it. But I also wonder if there is still the possibility that these cells in my CSF and I can co-exist, because maybe what I have is a weird thing on the cusp between autoimmune and malignant. Maybe we could treat until the cows come home and I'd still have funky lymphocytes in the CSF, and maybe it would be OK. I don't want you guys to treat my numbers and kill me in the process. Please keep that in mind when you talk to Sam after the flow results are back. And please keep me in the loop.

I was so relieved when Jack said he thought the visual trouble was from the steroids and not worsening lymphoma. I am paring down the faculties I absolutely need to live a happy life, and unfortunately vision is among them.

Laura

From: Laura
Sent: Friday, April 20, 2007 4:36 AM
To: Gerald
Subject: Help

Hi Gerald. We don't know each other well, since you just joined us at Memorial a few months ago, but I'm a long-standing fan of your cancer research. That's why I'm asking you for help.

This winter, I was diagnosed with disseminated lymphoma and started treatment with R-CHOP, intrathecal methotrexate, and high dose IV methotrexate at Memorial. A recent Omaya tap showed persistent atypical cells in my CSF. Phil, my oncologist, sent flow cytometry yesterday, which is pending. He says that if the atypical cells are lymphoma, we have to switch to stronger (and potentially more toxic) chemo.

Can you look at my lymphoma cells and design a targeted drug that would destroy my lymphoma cells and not kill the rest of me? I know you've been successful using this approach before in non-lymphoma cancers. I love my family more than you can imagine, and I'd like to have the chance to grow older with my husband and watch our kids grow up. I know that this kind of research can take years, and I may not have that kind of time.

As cancer doctors, we're trained to accept dying as a part of life. Now that I'm on the other side, I see how hard it is to stare death in the face and confront the possibility of leaving the people you love. I realize that my request is enormous (if not impossible), but if anyone can do it, it's you.

Laura

From: Laura
Sent: Saturday, April 21, 2007 7:25 AM
To: Jennifer
Subject: Movie

Dearest Jen,

I can see that you really read my emails—you rattled off a list of the people who make up the cast of characters of my life as if you had been there living it with me (which you are, in spirit!). I'm also glad you don't think my outburst traumatized my kids for life. That helps me a lot, coming from you.

You'll be delighted to hear that yesterday (Friday) was much better than Thursday! It started in the morning. The super was coming up to meet with David about the terrace and the bathroom. Nate thought that if I saw Jesus again I would explode, so he wanted to make sure that I wouldn't have any contact with the super. He told me that when the super comes, I should either go into another room or leave the apartment. He refused to go to school until David promised him to make sure that I did one or the other. Emma had already left, so I went into Emma's bathroom to take a shower, and stayed there with the door closed until David came in and told me that the super was gone.

Apparently it went well with the super. Jesus told David that they would finish the terrace within the week, and that the painters were coming in an hour to work on the bathroom. Jesus also told David that he has a prayer group, and he would like to bring his three friends over to pray for me. So I have to set a date to have the super's praying buddies make a house call!

I wanted to leave before the painters got there, because I knew it would make me upset. Luckily I had a good place to go. My friend Terri, an oncologist who makes documentaries about people living with cancer, had asked me to be in a film she was making called "The Physician as Patient," and she was filming that day. I had to pick the right clothes for the movie. I ended up wearing a muted purple silk shirt, a patterned multicolored yellow and purple skirt that I bought in St. Johns once on a Caribbean vacation, and a sweater in a combination of gold and purple. The most important decision, of course, was the hat. I picked a hat called the Butterfly, which is a soft mauve crown with medium brim and a muted gold silk organza butterfly-shaped bow.

To kill the time between 9 am and the movie shoot at 11:30 am, I went to our new clinical offices at 61st St. I wrote you when I saw the bare suite, but I haven't been back since everybody moved in. They moved offices when I was just starting treatment. I've had many prior office moves in the hospital and previously I've always packed and moved myself, meticulously labeling every box with books, journals, articles, and other items. This time, I didn't pack or move a single thing. I delegated it all to Lea, who did a spectacular job. She had even hung my pictures on the walls, so it really seemed like my office. And the windows that I was so excited about when I saw them for the first time—Jen, they actually open! And I look right at a huge sign that says Bed, Bath, and Beyond. The office is about twice the size of my previous radiology office, and the sun streams in through the windows.

Around 11:00 I left to go to the St. Regis Hotel, on 5th Avenue and 55th St. The hotel has an ornate lobby with lots of gold trim. I asked at the front desk where Terri was making the film. They told me the suite and I went up. When I entered the suite, they had just finished filming an 81-year-old doctor who had previously had head and neck cancer and now had prostate cancer. I chatted with him and his wife for awhile. Then the couple left and they set up for me.

The make-up part was a riot. I had blush, some kind of powder, and lipstick that I borrowed from Emma, but since I never wear make-up, I didn't know how to put them on. Terri and I went in front of the mirror in the bathroom, a room that is bigger than my entire apartment, and she applied the makeup to my face. She is absolutely meticulous—things had to be exactly balanced on both sides—it was like having Monk as your make-up artist! Emma's lipstick was too orange for me, so I did a trick that the cameraman from India suggested. There was a bowl of raspberries in the room, so I rubbed some raspberries on my lips to make them red. Apparently that is how the queens in India do it, so I guess now I have the qualifications to apply for a job as an Indian Queen.

The filming was done in the living room of the hotel suite, with overstuffed chairs, huge picture windows, and cut lilies in the background. It was a little hot in the room so they put on the air conditioning. I sat in the chair and I was wired up so tightly with mikes that I probably couldn't have escaped if I had wanted to. The film crew was two guys: Chris was in charge of the camera and Alex was in charge of sound. They were very friendly and joked around to try to put me at ease.

When it was time to start, Terri sat in the chair opposite me and asked questions. I got to tell a lot of my stories (although I left out the one about the panties and the brain surgery) and we talked about stuff I haven't really fully articulated in my mind (eg do you believe in life after death, do you believe in God, etc.). She asked questions about whether I got nervous waiting for test results, and I said not really. It's interesting that I said that—in the moment I completely forgot how terrified I am waiting for the results of the Omaya tap to see if the CSF has cleared. I guess the mind compartmentalizes. I had to take a couple of nausea pills to get through the filming. Afterwards, we went to a little outdoor plaza nearby to take some still photos.

Later, I met my friend Karen for tea. She's a breast imager from California and was in New York to visit her daughter. I've always admired her, because she does terrific work while still managing to keep her priorities straight. If she's invited to give a talk and she has family plans, she will do the family stuff and blow off the meeting. Her daughter is a sophomore at Columbia, studying Hispanic Studies and Human Rights. After tea, we walked back to my apartment and met up with her daughter. I took them for a walk on the boardwalk by the East River, and then I brought them home and introduced them to Emma and Nate. They left before dinnertime.

I was afraid to look in the bathroom until David got home, because I knew if I saw the fungus again I would lose it. When David came home, we looked at the bathroom together. Jen, it was a miracle. Those painters had scraped everything down to the bone, it was pure white, and the fungus was GONE. So it was worth it. One less thing trying to kill me.

That's all for now. Today I'm going to St. Patrick's cathedral to light candles with Cindy.

Love
Laura

From: Laura
Sent: Saturday, April 21, 2007 9:56 PM
To: Jennifer
Subject: Lighting candles

Hi Jen. Cindy and I met this afternoon at St. Patrick's cathedral, as planned. It was a gray day, lightly drizzling when I got there. I was wearing a black hat called the Lachlan, which has a square crown, medium brim bucket, and knot trim, in a soft waterproof fabric. The hat was perfect for the rain outside, but was hot in the church, so once we were inside, I took off the hat and put on my Monk cap, which I had stuffed into my purse.

I had never been inside St. Patrick's before. It was like a European cathedral. Incredibly high ceilings, ornate gold everywhere, and stained glass windows in vibrant colors with light shining through. When you come in, there's a marble water fountain on your left, which Cindy said has holy water. I asked whether you drink it, and she said no, you bless yourself with it. Apparently you are allowed to bring a bottle with you and take some holy water for the road. I dipped my fingertips in it and sprinkled some on my head and shoulders.

We walked around the church. In the center were multiple long wooden benches. At the periphery were statues of saints, each enclosed by a couple of marble steps and a small fence. A little plaque near each saint explained the name of the saint and what the saint stood for. To your lower left as you looked at the saint, there were bins that had many round, relatively flat, unlit candles. More centrally, there were several rows of small glass cups, some with lit candles inside. The round candles fit perfectly into the glass cups. There was another bin full of wooden sticks, thinner and longer than chopsticks.

If you want to light a candle to a saint, you pick up an unlit candle, gently pull up the wick so that it's standing rather than flat against the wax, and drop the candle into an empty glass cup. You take one of the wooden sticks, put the tip in the flame of one candle, and use that to light your candle. After the candle is lit, you can blow out the flame on your stick or extinguish it by putting it directly into this thin rectangular planter full of dirt. We enjoyed putting it into the dirt, because it made a satisfying little hissing sound as the fire went out.

Cindy recognized the saints, although I didn't know most of them. I read all the cards. I was looking for a saint for 47-year-old women with lymphoma. None of the saints exactly fit the bill, but I was able to find saints for the sick, the dying, the departed, and people in need. I figured close enough, and lit the candles. After we had walked halfway around the church, there was a quiet area with several benches separate from the main central portion of the Cathedral. From the benches, there was a beautiful view of the stained glass windows and an altar at the front. We sat there quietly for awhile. Then we got up, looped around the other side of the church lighting candles for a few more saints, and left the cathedral.

Although it was near dusk, the light outside glared after the dim of the church. It was also jarring to come out of the cathedral and immediately be inundated by the bustle and commercialism of New York City, including an Armani Emporium right across the street. Cindy and I didn't talk much. It had stopped drizzling by then. We walked back to the Upper East Side, where Cindy had parked her car. We gave each other a hug. She got into her car and I hopped a cab back to my apartment.

I know that lighting candles in a cathedral is an odd experience for a nice Jewish girl. I'm not a born again Christian (or any kind of Christian). When I was growing up, my parents shared a strong sense of Jewish cultural identity but weren't religious—my dad used to say that many atrocities in world history were committed in the name of God. But confronting the fact that I might die makes me look for answers and spiritual solace wherever I can find them. I need to connect with other people, with the universe, and with what, if anything, is beyond it.

Tomorrow, back to earth. Emma and I have tickets to see a Broadway show.

Love
Laura

From: Laura
Sent: Sunday, April 22, 2007 6:18 AM
To: Q
Subject: Invitation

Dearest Q,

I'm writing this letter to invite you, Steve, Nick, and Ben to our "re-wedding." David and I are going to celebrate our 25th anniversary by getting unofficially married again. We're hoping to have the celebration on Sunday June 10 (the actual anniversary is June 13), either on our terrace if it's ready or in Carl Schurz Park if it's not. It will be very simple—just the eight of us (no rabbi or other officiating person) and we'll read something out loud and give each other a hug and a kiss and that's it. Afterwards we'll have dinner. Can you join us?

Love
Laura

From: Laura
Sent: Sunday, April 22, 2007 11:25 PM
To: Jennifer
Subject: Spring Awakening

Hi Jen. I had a wonderful day with Emma today. It was sunny and warm outside, maybe the first real spring day we've had so far. I wore a hat called the Olivia, which was a fabric cloche with piped crown and hand-rolled roses in a luscious lime green.

Emma came with me to drop off some dry cleaning, and then we went shopping. We went to Eileen Fisher, and bought some comfortable pants with an elastic waist in beige and black. I also got a button-down sweater that doesn't pull over my head. All my clothes have to be easy now. No energy to spend on snaps and zippers and buckles. We also got a great jacket for Emma from the Petites section. Then we went next door to Le Sportsac, and Emma helped me choose a pouch I can use to organize all the stuff I carry with me now (Meds, iPod, anti-nausea pills, pencils, toothbrush, toothpaste, numbing spray, and anesthetic cream).

After a quick lunch, Emma and I went to see "Spring Awakening," a Broadway musical about a young girl's coming of age. We've been listening to the CD, but hadn't seen the show yet. Emma and I have been seeing musicals together for years. I love our excursions. I've always been a big fan of musicals, and the boys never want to go; David and Nate both believe that people should not spontaneously burst into song. It's great to spend time with Emma—she's such a bundle of joy and energy. Any experience is more fun if Emma is there to share it.

I remember our first mother-daughter outing to the theater more than a decade ago. Emma was three, and I had gotten tickets for us to see the ballet at Lincoln Center. All around us were mother-daughter couples, including one couple next to us with a mom in her 50s and a daughter in her 30s who have apparently been coming to Lincoln Center together for more than twenty years. Emma was very excited at the beginning of the show but when I turned to talk to her as the curtain rose at Intermission, I saw she was fast asleep. The most expensive nap in history.

We loved Spring Awakening. There were young actors we'd never seen before and the music had a strange combination of dissonance and consonance as well as a mix of styles including classic show-tune, gospel, and rock. Afterwards, I got Emma a Spring Awakening t shirt and the script of the play from which the musical was adapted (although the story was primarily an excuse for the music). We took a cab home and the four of us had dinner together. Nate and David went out to a jazz club. Emma and I listened to the music from the show and fell asleep before the CD ended.

Love
Laura

From: Laura
Sent: Monday, April 23, 2007 11:59 AM
To: Peter
Subject: Flow cytometry

Hi Peter. I had a repeat Omaya tap to see if there are still lymphoma cells in my CSF. Can you give me a buzz at x7289 to discuss the results of the flow cytometry? I gather this is the critical test.
Thanks!

Laura

From: Laura
To: Phil
Sent: Mon Apr 23 12:07 AM
Subject: Go with the flow

I talked to Peter about the CSF flow results and he said it's negative for lambda or kappa clonal excess. Apparently that means there's no lymphoma in the CSF! That's one for the home team.
After Cycle 3, we have to confirm that the cells are clear in the LP. I'll set it up.

Laura

From: Laura
Sent: Monday, April 23, 2007 9:45 PM
To: Jennifer
Subject: Good news

Hi Jen. Thanks for your note. I know how hard it is to find a new nanny. I wish I could launch a Philadelphia spin-off of our Nanny Resource list-serve for you and find you a perfect nanny. I'll ask Carmen if she knows of any nannies in Philly.

I got some good news today—the flow cytometry on my CSF showed no clonal excess! In English, that means that the funky lymphocytes in my CSF are probably NOT lymphoma. I need to confirm that finding with another lumbar puncture (LP, or spinal tap), to make absolutely sure that the CSF is clear, but this raises my chances considerably. This result is just what I was hoping for, and I'm glad about it, but I can't completely rejoice until we confirm the results with an LP, which will happen after I finish this round of chemo.

Yes, I'm being admitted tomorrow for more high-dose IV methotrexate. I'll probably go home Sunday. I hope I get admitted back to M8. They were so nice to me the last time.

Have to pack for my admission. My next emails will be from the hospital.

Love
Laura

From: Laura
Sent: Tuesday, April 24, 2007 9:49 PM

To: Maureen
Subject: Thank you

Hi Maureen. Thank you for leading Athena tonight! I already hear through the grapevine that you did a fantastic job. Can't wait to hear the details.

Love
Laura

From: Laura
Sent: Wednesday, April 25, 2007 1:21 AM
To: Gerald
Subject: Never mind

Hi Gerald. I'm writing to apologize for the desperate middle-of-the-night email I sent you a couple of days ago. I'm glad I got your autoreply that you're out of town with limited email access. When I sent the email, it looked like my lymphoma wasn't responding to the chemo and I got scared. Luckily, the news this week was great. My CSF is clear—no lymphoma! So we're both off the hook for now. Hopefully, when you get back, you'll read both of these emails at the same time and know not to worry.

In this place where we spend most of our lives fighting cancer, it's good to have you on our team. I won't be shy to write if I need you again.

Best wishes
Laura

From: Laura
Sent: Wednesday, April 25, 2007 2:54 AM
To: Jennifer
Subject: Second admission

Hi Jen. I'm sorry you're short of breath. You're so petite, the baby occupies a substantial portion of you, and when your diaphragm tries to descend to allow the lungs to expand, your belly is telling your diaphragm "stay away from me!" Don't worry, this too will pass, and soon you will have your beautiful baby boy. I can't wait to meet him!

Yesterday I was re-admitted for more IV methotrexate. Wearing my Monk cap, I went up to the 4th floor to see Phil in the Clinic. Cindy met me there—I wasn't sure if they were going to give me another intrathecal chemo today or not. After I had my fingerstick, they called us into the office. Phil told me that since my flow cytometry was negative, I don't need to get more intrathecal chemo for the time being. HOORAY! He said that after the third round of IV chemo I'll get an LP as well as repeat MRIs of the spine and brain, and then we'll discuss with Sam whether I need more intrathecal chemo at all.

I went to the Admitting office, and finally I was admitted back to M8. It's a different room, but still fine. The computer has this weird soft rubber keyboard which takes a little getting used to, but the layout is normal (QWERTYUIOP etc.). I already had multiple visitors, including one who brought me flowers which I'm allowed to have today because my white blood cell count is still OK. When your white cell count falls after chemo, they don't allow you to have flowers because they could be a source of infection.

146

The nurse "accessed the port" after I sprayed it, and hooked me up to the pump on the IV. The IV pump follows me everywhere, beeping whenever it's unplugged. They started the bicarbonate drip and gave me the premeds. The methotrexate started at 7:30 pm and ran for four hours, so it was done at 11:30 pm. Now I'm getting more bicarb. I get hydrated all day tomorrow, and then I get the leukovorin rescue starting 24 hours after the methotrexate began. So far so good.

Terri is busy editing her movie on "The Physician as Patient." She'll present it at the annual meeting of the American Society of Clinical Oncology (ASCO) in June.

I'm getting sleepy. While I go to sleep, I'm going to listen to Yo-Yo Ma and Emanuel Ax doing the Brahms E Minor Sonata for Cello and Piano that you and I used to play together (Allegro non troppo, Allegretto Quasi Menuetto—Trio, and Allegro). Usually I'm asleep before the end of the first movement.

Love
Laura

From: Laura
Sent: Wednesday, April 25, 2007 3:32 PM
To: Women Faculty
Subject: Athena lives

To Our Guests at Athena last night:

I'm writing to thank you for coming to Athena last night. It means so much to me that Athena lives even when I can't be there—it means that our group is self-sustaining. I especially want to thank Maureen for hosting the meeting while I was getting chemo. And I actually did join in the toast you had for me—I just did it with methotrexate instead of white wine. I've now received 9 of 18 chemos (halfway)!

I'll beat this. You can't keep a good woman down.

Laura

From: Laura
Sent: Wednesday, May 2, 2007 6:29 AM
To: Jennifer
Subject: Tales from inside the house

Hi Jen. Sorry for my long silence. I had to focus on getting through my admission. But things are good, and I have many stories to tell you to catch up!

First, about the admission. I wrote to you that the high-dose methotrexate went fine, and the rest was also pretty uneventful, fluids and peeing. They put a plastic container euphemistically called a "hat" in the toilet that collects all the urine so that it can be measured, and they track my Intake and Output (Is and Os). The system is imperfect—they carefully monitor every cubic centimeter (cc) of fluid that I get IV, but then they ask me how much I drank, and I have no idea, so I just make up a number. No matter when they ask how much I've had to drink, I look at them confidently and say, "200 cc."

They take my vital signs (pulse, temperature, blood pressure) every six hours. I had a running joke with the nurses' aides about the impressiveness of my vital signs. When the team came by to round in the morning I told them that I had the best vital signs on the floor. Some of the nurses' aides thought it was hysterical, and others seemed puzzled by me. Maybe some of the M8 patients getting bone marrow transplant who are in the hospital for weeks at a time get a little depressed and don't talk much to the aides.

Apparently the fellow on my team heard me brag that I had the best vital signs on the floor, and when she presented me at lymphoma rounds to the other doctors, she described me (in good humor) as a competitive overachiever. A friend of mine who is a lymphoma doc and attends lymphoma rounds told me what the fellow said. So the next day, when the fellow came to see me at rounds, I told her, "I hear that in rounds you called me a competitive overachiever... I just hope you realize that if I am a competitive overachiever, that I am the best competitive overachiever on the floor!" We laughed.

I had terrific nurses. My day nurse was usually Trish, and my night nurse was a wonderful person named (of all things) Jen! It's amazing how much the nurses affect your hospital experience. The doctors breeze in, glance at your chart, ask a couple of questions, listen to your heart and lungs for two minutes, and then disappear into doctorland to write notes and orders. When you need a Tylenol at 3 am or something hurts, it's the nurses who come. I'm amazed at how softly the nurses can tiptoe into your room in the wee hours of the morning and do what needs to be done without waking you up.

Guess what—Nate grew up! I never knew that I would be able to identify the precise date when he grew up, but it was Thursday, April 26, 2007. It was around 7:30 in the morning, and David had dropped by to have breakfast with me in the hospital. He started coming to have breakfast with me most mornings when I was in the hospital, after he got the kids off to school. It was our time together. That morning, while David was visiting, I called Nate to tell him I was worried because he didn't seem to be doing much homework. Over the phone, I told him that I was concerned that he would jeopardize what he has spent three years in high school trying to achieve.

Nate calmly explained that he had already spoken to all of his teachers. He had discussed every single subject, reviewing what assignments he has, which ones he has to do, which ones he can skip, which papers he can hand in late, etc. Nate said he wanted to be in control of his schoolwork, which showed a great deal of insight and self-awareness; he can't control my cancer, but he can control his work. He said that he hadn't told me because he didn't want to burden me, but that he's taking care of his work and he asked that I respect that. This was no teenager; he was mature and rational. I hung up the phone, turned to David, and said, "He's an adult."

I had a lot of visitors. It's nice to see people, but sometimes it got a little out of control. It's hardest when four people who don't know each other come at once. For my next admission, I'm going to get a guest book and have people sign in and make comments at the door.

I narrowly dodged a blood transfusion. I was anemic to begin with (my hemoglobin was 8 point something; normal is 12), and then when they hydrated the hell out of me, my hemoglobin went down to 7.5 (basically they diluted my hemoglobin, a process called "hemodilution"). I had agreed to be transfused if it went below 7 but really didn't want a transfusion if it wasn't essential. So I claimed I had just become a Jehova's witness ("Jehova was just here! I witnessed Him!") and talked them into giving me darbopoietin, an injection that helps your bone marrow produce more red blood cells. Thank God I avoided the transfusion. The more they do to you, the greater the chances that something will go wrong—or, as we used to say in internship, the more you stay, the more you stay. My hemoglobin started to come up, so it worked out OK.

During this admission, I continued doing laps around the nurses' station while listening to my iPod and pushing my IV pole. At first I counted the number of laps, but then I started just doing an hour every morning, before I shower. Just turn on Stevie Wonder (At the Close of a Century, Disc 2) and I'm ready to rock and roll. I listen to a lot of classical music in the room (this time I especially enjoyed Mozart Violin Sonatas with Hilary Hahn and Natalie Zhu), but when I'm walking I go for more popular stuff.

I was discharged before noon on Saturday. David came to pick me up with his mom, who was visiting from California. We had brunch with the kids at home, toasted bagels and unsalted nova and cream cheese and fresh orange juice, one of my favorite New York traditions. After she left, I went to pick up new prescription glasses and I can see! It's miraculous.

Re the plan for chemo etc.—I'm getting IV R-CHOP again tomorrow. After my next admission, I'll be done with the third cycle of chemo and they'll do restaging tests.

Love
Laura

From: Laura
Sent: Saturday, May 5, 2007 2:56 AM
To: Jennifer
Subject: Seeing the light

Dearest Jen,

I've reached a new phase in this cancer thing. I've already finished 10/18 planned doses of chemo, so I'm past the halfway mark. I can see the light at the end of the tunnel.

I enjoyed my laps around the nurses' station during my last admission so much that I decided to try walking on the beautiful boardwalk overlooking the East River by my house, called John Finley walk, in Carl Schurz Park. I enter the Park at 88th Street, right next to Gracie Mansion, which is the Mayor's mansion (although Bloomberg doesn't live there, because apparently his own apartment is even nicer!). When you walk on the boardwalk, you can see a majestic view of the river, boats, Roosevelt Island, the Triborough Bridge, light, and sky. A moderately paced walk from one side of the boardwalk to the other takes ten minutes, so you can do three complete laps back and forth in one hour. If you're very ambitious, you can go down the staircase on one side of the boardwalk and walk further downtown as far as the East 60s, and then come back.

For the past several days, I've been doing this walk for an hour each morning, wearing my iPod, listening to different music every day (The Supremes, the soundtrack of Wicked, Carole King, James Taylor). It's fun! There's a whole culture out there in the mornings, with runners, walkers, newspaper-readers, bike-riders, stroller-pushers, etc. I particularly love seeing the people play with their dogs in a special fenced off-area. The dogs hang out on one side and the people on the other, like it's a big cocktail party. The other day a man sat on a bench reading the paper, and next to him was his large long-legged dog. The dog's front legs were on the pavement, but his butt and hind legs were up on the bench—he sat on the bench like a person! I wish I'd had my digital camera.

Today I went to my 61st Street office. I read through snail mail, which included more cancer presents, and emails. For the book I'm writing, I'm trying to decide whether to include just the emails I send, which are mostly to you, or whether I should also include emails I get from other people. I've gotten some wonderful and supportive emails, and it may be nice to include them, because one take-home message I'd like to give people is that if you reach out to people, sometimes they are there for you in wonderful ways. If I do include other people's emails, I'll let the authors of those emails read the book and ask their permission to let me use the emails as written.

Tonight David and I had a date. We went to see Cassandra Wilson at the Blue Note. She is a wonderful jazz singer who doesn't do a lot of club dates in the States anymore. I wore a new black sleeveless dress, a turquoise sweater, pearls, and a hat called the Lucy, which is a black weave with a soft silk silver bow. The music and dinner were fabulous but we were crushed in like sardines. It was the first time David and I went out to hear jazz together since his birthday party. I looked at David during the music and pictured him at jazz clubs over the years, starting when he was a kid in the Bronx and too young to get into the clubs so he would listen by the door.

I figured out how this lymphoma will behave. I'm going to go into remission with the chemotherapy, and will transform this acute threat on my life into a nice chronic disease for which I'll have to take pills and have follow-up tests. Every few years I will recur, because that's what lymphomas do. When I recur, they'll blast me with chemo, which I'll tolerate remarkably well, and I'll go into another remission. As time goes by, they'll do more research; the chemo will get better and the remissions will be longer. And I could percolate around like this for twenty years, or maybe longer, until one day the recurrence will get me or I'll be hit by a bus or something entirely different. And maybe I'll outlive everybody else, and be looking for someone to whom I can send emails at 2 am. Good plan?

How are you today? Do you feel like the baby will come any minute now? When is the actual due date again?

Love
Laura

From: Laura
Sent: Saturday, May 5, 2007 1:27 PM
To: Mike
Subject: Your hat

Hi Mike. I guess Mel told you about my lymphoma. How wonderful that you sent me two hats! I bought 15 hats at the beginning of chemo, and since then people have been sending me hats as presents (usually baseball caps). Until today, I had 28 hats; your hats are #29 and #30. At this rate, I'll be able to get through the rest of my chemo and never wear any hat more than three times!

I'm impressed that you wore one of the hats during a New Year's Day Alcatraz swim, and the other when you finished the Ironman World Championship Triatholon in Hawaii. I love the card, "Wear these be victorious."

Keep those prayers coming. If God hears from a rogue like you, he'll know something is up that he has to take seriously. Since you're Greek, maybe you should pray to a Greek God. Let's get Zeus on board.

I'm doing great. I'm more than half done with the chemo, and I started walking about an hour every day on this gorgeous boardwalk by the East River, right next to my house. One of these days (after my white cells come back), I mayl jump in the water and become a Polar Bear like you

I'm writing a book about being a doctor and a patient, and it's more than half done. I was going to call it *Both Sides Now,* like the Judy Collins song. Unfortunately, there are already about a million books with that title. These books include, but are not limited to, *Both Sides Now: A Twenty-Five Year Encounter with Arabs and Israelis, Both Sides Now: The Story of School Desegregation's Graduates, Both Sides Now: Living and Dying in San Francisco,* and, my personal favorite, *Both Sides Now: One Man's Journey through Womanhood.* I had to come up with another name. I've decided to call it *I Signed as the Doctor* because when they gave me the consent forms to sign for those god-awful procedures when treatment began, I kept forgetting I'm the patient, so I signed as the doctor!

We're already fantasizing about the post-chemo celebration vacation to Turks and Caicos in September. Blue sea, white sand, not a care in the world, and I hear I can bump into Donna Karan by the pool. But I'll be in the ocean snorkeling with fish in the reef.

Love to Sheila. Keep the faith.

Love
Laura

From: Laura
Sent: Saturday, May 5, 2007 3:13 PM
To: Jung-min
Subject: Hi! And a few things

Jung-min—are you at the American Roentgen Ray Society meeting today? I left you a message on your cell—I called for a few reasons:

1. Good luck! Your presentation will be fabulous.

2. Can you pick up an abstract book for me? If they give you a hard time, tell them it is for a colleague of yours with cancer who couldn't come to the meeting. And ask for it early in the week—by later in the week, they tend to disappear.

3. Who is the moderator of the scientific session at which you'll be presenting? Before the presentation starts, go up to the moderator, introduce yourself, and check out the podium. Make sure you know how to advance the slides or go back, how the pointer works, and where the timer is so you can pace yourself.

4. I've gotten multiple phone calls about you for recommendations for the various programs for which you're applying, and I tell them you are fabulous. But promise me you won't accept any offers until we talk. I want to give you my best advice when you have all the offers on the table.

You can call me back on my cell, email me, or call me at home. Which day is your talk, and when are you coming back? Are you staying at the meeting hotel? Are the accommodations OK? Do you know anyone at the meeting?

It is a beautiful day in New York today. I hope your trip was gentle and that you are having a wonderful time. Enjoy!

Love
Laura

From: Laura
Sent: Tuesday, May 8, 2007 4:10 AM

To: Jennifer
Subject: Baby?

Dearest Jen,

How are YOU? What is the status of Baby Boy Menell? When I didn't hear from you I thought you had the baby— what's going on? Can you email me your cell phone, home phone, and work phone numbers again? In my prednisone craze I can't find them. Otherwise, I'm doing great and will resume writing to you more regularly soon.

David and I saw the play "Inherit the Wind" on Broadway, and it was fantastic. It's funny how a play about evolution vs. creationism can be so relevant to current times. I'd been excited to see Brian Dennehy, but I was really blown away by Christopher Plummer. They were both amazing.

I miss you and love you very much, and wish you every joy in your new son, whenever he decides to make his debut.

Love
Laura

From: Laura
Sent: Saturday, May 19, 2007 10:44 AM
To: Jennifer
Subject: Third admission

Dearest Jen,

It's been awhile since I wrote you a good long letter, so here it comes. I'm an inpatient now, finishing up Cycle 3 of chemo with the high-dose IV methotrexate and leucovorin rescue. The chemo went fine on Thursday—no problems. I got admitted a little earlier than usual, so they started the chemo earlier, which made the schedule flow a little more smoothly.

I've been feeling good, in spite of my ongoing worry about the LP I'll have when this cycle of chemo is over. I'm walking laps around the nurses' station again with the iPod, but I miss the boardwalk. I had so many visitors during my last admission that this time I brought a guest book—you know, like they have at a country inn or someone's wedding? The guest book had a soft green cover and cream-colored paper, and I had bought it at Kate's Paperie. I invite my guests to sign in and make comments. I considered having a cover charge and a two-drink minimum, but apparently that violates hospital regulations.

Today I had tickets for Emma and me to see A Chorus Line that I had bought months ago, but since I'm still in the hospital, Emma invited a friend to go with her. It will be her first Broadway show without me. I hope they have fun.

So when is this baby going to appear? Keep me posted!

Love
Laura

From: Liberman, Laura/Radiology
Sent: Wednesday, May 23, 2007 1:27 PM
To: Jennifer
Subject: LP results

Hi Jen. I had my LP (lumbar puncture, or spinal tap) yesterday. The procedure is done by a neuroradiologist under fluoroscopy ("fluoro"), x-ray equipment that gives instantaneous images of your bones and other structures. You lie face down on a table, and then the table tilts so that your head is up and your feet are down, at an angle. The radiologist uses the fluoro to figure out exactly where to put the needle, usually between the 3rd and 4th of the five lumbar vertebrae (the back bones in the lower spine). My wonderful friend Hilda did the LP, and Sam came in person to deliver the fluid to the lab.

Today they got the results. There were only two white blood cells, down from 76, with no clonal excess. In English, that means no evidence of lymphoma! With the negative LP and the negative Omaya tap, we can say that the CSF is clear. I wish I could play the music from "I Will Survive," but that will make me feel like dancing, and I'm supposed to lie flat for several hours after the LP (I shouldn't even be sitting at the computer to write you this note, but I can't resist). I bought the DVD of "Dreamgirls," and Carmen and I are going to watch it together.

The baby is due any day now, right? You must be so excited. You'll finally get to meet your son!

Love
Laura

Chapter 12
More Birthdays

Savor celebrations.

From: Laura
Sent: Sunday, May 27, 2007 11:56 PM
To: Jennifer
Subject: Emma's birthday

Hi Jen. Today was Emma's 15th birthday. Since her birthday falls on Memorial Day weekend this year, we're having the party for her friends next week, but today we had the family celebration.

In the morning, we showered her with gifts—books and DVDs that we thought she'd like, as well as camera equipment (she has a passion for photography). We let her pick what meal she'd like to go out for, and what restaurant. She wanted me to take her to lunch at Candle 79, our favorite Vegan restaurant in the city. Then we went shopping together at her favorite stores—Urban Outfitters, American Apparel, H&M.

In the evening, we turned out the lights, gave her a cake with 16 candles, one of which was for good luck, and sang "Happy Birthday." I bought her the cake at Greenberg's, one of the best bakeries on the East Side of Manhattan, where I've been getting the kids their birthday cakes every year since they were old enough to eat chocolate. Emma's cake this year was pure chocolate—chocolate cake with chocolate frosting, and said "Happy Birthday Emma" in yellow icing on top.

As I watched Emma and Nate while we sang happy birthday, I thought about how different they are from each other.

Nate has always been cautious; he looks so much before he leaps that sometimes he doesn't get around to the leaping part. Emma, on the other hand, is absolutely fearless. When Nate and I used to cross the street when he was young, he would hold my hand, and ask, "Is it OK, Mom?" If Emma saw something interesting on the other side of the street, she would have dashed across if I hadn't been holding her hand tightly. Since Nate is older and more cautious, he always looks out for his sister, and has since she was a baby and tried to put seashells into her mouth at the beach.

Emma is the most extroverted member of our family. When she was two and a half, we signed her up for a program called Discovery that was held for about three hours twice a week. On the first day, the other kids all had trouble separating. Emma looked in the room, saw that there were art supplies, and said "Bye, Mom!" She has always been like a Pied Piper for other kids—when she went to the park, all of the other kids wanted to play with Emma. She has a way of relating to kids of any age—whether they are younger, older, or the same age, she manages to find common ground.

Emma's birthday today made me think back to her other birthdays, like the one when she was in third grade. I had taken a vacation day from work so that we could celebrate after school. She had the mildest case of pink-eye that day, so the school nurse wanted to send her home. Emma was initially sad to be kicked out of school on her birthday, but when I picked her up, I told her, "Emma, don't worry. We'll shop 'till we drop!" As it turned out, after about three stores she was still bursting with energy but I was exhausted. She gleefully told me, "We shopped until YOU dropped, Mommy!"

I can't believe that Emma will be going to sleepaway camp in a few weeks. I'll miss her. She's like a bundle of sunshine—it's impossible to be sad around Emma. When she goes, there is this big hole that's impossible to fill. But she loves camp, and at least they cut it down from eight weeks to six. The first time Emma went to sleepaway camp, a woman in my building asked me how I was doing. I said, "My daughter just went to sleepaway camp for the first time, and I miss her." The woman said to me authoritatively, "When my son went to college, I cried for two weeks. Then, I moved into his closets!" She was saying that in New York, it's OK when a child leaves, because look how much you gain in closet space!

How are you doing? Do you think the baby will come today? Then he and Emma would have the same birthday!

Love
Laura

From: Laura
Sent: Wednesday, May 30, 2007 5:49 AM
To: Jennifer
Subject: Great news

Dearest Jen,

Congratulations on Benjamin Matthew! You've used two of my favorite boys' names in the whole world. I love the name Benjamin, whether it's Ben or Benny. Like Nate, he'll probably declare himself as one or the other.

How did Sophie react when you brought home her new brother? I'll never forget bringing Emma home from the hospital. Nate greeted her at the door with a photo album and called her "Baby." He showed her pictures of the people in our family and tried to teach her their names. He also showed her pictures from a trip to the zoo, and explained, "Look, Baby, here's a peacock!" Emma couldn't even hold her head up, much less scrutinize the photographs. But Nate was undeterred. At dinner that night, he offered Emma a forkful of his food and asked, "Baby, want some steak?" I had to explain that Emma was too young to eat steak, that so far all she could handle was milk, and that we would have to teach her lots of things.

I got some great news this week. After I finished the third cycle of chemo, they repeated the spine MRI and the CT scan, and they were negative! The spine MRI showed that the 3 cm tumor that I used to have in my upper spinal cord is GONE, and the CT showed that the lymph nodes are smaller. So chemo works! I don't need any more intrathecal chemo injected into my head, but I need three more months of IV chemo.

I thought I was supposed to get R-CHOP yesterday but apparently I'm getting it Thursday. That changes my chemo schedule in a way that means I get to be home on our 25th wedding anniversary. David and I are going to have a little ceremony where we renew our vows on our terrace, either that day or on the weekend after I'm discharged. It's not going to be fancy—just the four of us, and maybe some close family friends.

The vows we're going to read are from a list of promises we wrote to each other when I followed David to New York for medical school. It was so long ago we didn't even have a word processor—we typed it on our old Smith-Corona typewriter. I looked at it today for the first time in years. The paper is yellowed and crinkly, and there's a typo with a hand-written correction. The promises were pretty astute, though, especially considering that we were kids—eg "We won't let our perceptions of each other's parents blur our perceptions of each other" and "We won't let each other be lonely." And then there's one that is unoriginal but still one of my favorites: "We will take care of each other in sickness and in health." I'm thinking, damn, I'm glad we put that in!

Have fun with the new baby. It's an amazing time. And take advantage of any opportunity to spend time with Sophie, who was just "dethroned" by her new sibling—it'll mean the world to both of you.

Love
Laura

From: Laura
Sent: Saturday, June 2, 2007 4:04 AM
To: Jennifer
Subject: The Prednisone Diaries, Revisited

Dearest Jen,

And here we go again—back on Prednisone! At least I can count on writing in the wee hours of the morning for five days a month. I'm in the midst of Cycle 4 out of 6 cycles of IV R-CHOP. I can't believe I have only 4 more chemos left (2 IV RCHOPS and 2 high-dose IV methotrexates).

We're busy making preparations for Emma's 15th birthday party, which will be on our roof tomorrow night. Since her birthday at the end of May usually falls on Memorial Day weekend, we generally have her party in early June.

Please let me know how the bris went, and keep me posted about Benjamin and Sophie and Jim and nursing and sleeping (or lack thereof) and everything else in your life that you want to share.

Much love always
Laura

From: Laura
Sent: Monday, June 4, 2007 3:29 AM
To: Jennifer
Subject: Emma's 15th birthday party

Hi Jen. Last night was Emma's 15th birthday party with her friends. We had it on the roof of our building, so we could use the rooftop swimming pool, surrounding terrace with lounge chairs, other outside areas, and the room with the ping-pong table. I had heard that there was going to be a thunderstorm, in which case they would have either stayed in the ping pong room or gone downstairs to another party room in our building. Luckily, though, the weather held out, and they stayed on the roof.

Emma wanted to keep it simple—pizza, chips, soda, brownies—music from the iPoD—dancing—ping pong— swimming. Even with that plan, there was a lot to prepare. We got the food and the drinks (sodas and water), paper plates, and plastic utensils. We cut up carrots and celery for appetizers and Emma made a delicious dip (she is truly a fabulous cook). Emma made a playlist of the music she wanted to play. Three friends came early to help set up.

The party was a big success. One guy had forgotten to bring his bathing suit, and Nate generously went up to the roof to lend him one of his prior bathing suits, which fit the guy perfectly. We provided towels for everyone who wanted to swim. When you have parties by the pool in our building, you are obliged to use a lifeguard from the service that generally works at the pool, so the lifeguard was there. The party was from 7-11 pm. Since it's already starting to stay light a little later, there was about an hour and a half of light before it got dark, and then they turned on the lights upstairs, which made the pool glow an inviting turquoise blue.

After the party, David, Emma, and I cleaned up. There were a few dishes to wash, and we had to throw away a lot of used paper goods. Emma was happy, bubbling over with excitement about the night. She had a stack of presents but decided that she'd open them in the morning.

Once when I was quizzing Nate on Spanish vocabulary to prepare for a test, we came across the word "Quincenara," which is the celebration for a girl's 15ᵗʰ birthday. I guess the Latina tradition is to celebrate sweet 15 instead of sweet 16. Emma had a wonderful Quincenara.

Love
Laura

From: Junior Faculty Council (JFC)
Sent: Wednesday, June 13, 2007 10:39 AM
To: Faculty Nominated for Mentoring Award
Subject: MH 2007 Mentoring Award Nomination

Dear Colleagues,

We recently announced a new Memorial Hospital Award for Excellence in Mentoring. On behalf of the Junior Faculty Council, we are pleased to inform you that you have been nominated by a Junior Faculty member as an Outstanding Mentor.

We received many outstanding nominations and we thank you all for your contributions to mentoring. The recipient of this award for 2007 will be announced at the JFC Town Meeting, Tuesday, June 19th in room M-107, 12:30.

We hope that you can join us in celebrating this important achievement.

Congratulations,
JFC

From: Laura
Sent: Saturday, June 16, 2007 10:15 AM
To: Jennifer
Subject: Wedding anniversary

Dearest Jen,

When I read your note about how tough it can be with the second baby, I remember back to when Emma was born. It is much harder after the second than the first, because there are two tugging at your energy and attention. That was when I considered going part-time, and almost did it. It wasn't until Emma was about six months old that I felt I was kind of hitting my stride again a little bit. It's good that you had a baby nurse for awhile. How is the nanny doing? Are you getting to spend any time with just Sophie?

Time is going by so quickly now. Wednesday was our 25th wedding anniversary. We renewed our vows on the terrace with the kids. It was just the four of us because the Berkowitzes couldn't come. I wore a white lace shirt, a colorful print skirt, and a white hat, and David wore a suit. We alternated back and forth reading our promises to each other, with the sweeping East River and the Tri-Borough Bridge as the backdrop. Then we gave each other gifts. David got me a new ring, with a plain gold band sprinkled with tiny diamonds. I loved it because it seemed to be a perfect metaphor for our marriage: multiple tiny sparkling moments that add up to a lifetime of being together. I gave him an engraved watch. Afterwards, we asked the kids what they wanted for dinner and ordered out for Thai food. That's a 25-year marriage.

On Thursday, I was admitted to the hospital for my second-to-last round of inpatient chemo. Everything moved slowly that day. I had a 9 am appointment with Phil. I was very anemic and he wanted to give me a shot of darbopoeiten, but that had to be ordered from the pharmacy, so I waited until 11 am. Then I went to Admitting, but I had left my hospital card at Phil's office, so I had to go back and get it, and while I was there they wanted to change an appointment, which took time. I got back to Admitting at almost 12, and it was afternoon by the time I got to M8. Then they had to do a blood test for electrolytes and wait for the results; it took forever to start the bicarb drip.

I usually need to be on the drip about 4 hours to alkalinize my urine pH above 7.5. Only after the urine pH is high enough do they order the methotrexate, which then has to be mixed and delivered from Pharmacy. I didn't start the methotrexate until 8 pm, and it's a 4-hour infusion. Once I get the methotrexate, then 24 hours later I get leucovorin "rescue," and continue to get leucovorin every 6 hours as long as I'm here. So it means that my schedule for the leucovorin is 8-2-8-2 (which means I have to get up for vital signs at midnight and then they hang the leucovorin at 2 am). The first night I only slept about two hours, but I got a little nap on Friday, so I was OK.

David came in the morning on Friday and we had breakfast together, which was nice. Lots of visitors on Friday, including Cindy and our wonderful technologists with whom I've become very close over the years—Youngduk, Indira, Anita, and Joanna—and they came with frozen yogurt! I brought my guest book back with me this time and most of my visitors signed it and wrote in it, like they did during my previous admission.

Emma came by herself later in the day and did my nails in a beautiful sparkling white. Nate joined her, and then David came. We all hung out together until they went home around 8:45, and I went to bed. Slept until 4 am, woke up drenched (I have night sweats), got up and showered and changed, and then felt so awake I walked my laps around the nurses' station. Then I came back to my room and napped about two hours, until 8 o'clock when Kathy, my nurse, came in to hang the 8 am leucovorin and give me my morning meds.

They've decided I need a total of 16 chemos, not 18 as they originally thought, and I've had 13 out of those 16 chemos already. If everything goes according to plan, I need three more chemos after this: two outpatient IV R-CHOPS and one more admission for IV methotrexate. My last chemo will be at the end of July, less than two months from now. In August, I'll have another re-staging work-up, including an MRI and a bone marrow. I'm trying to figure out how I'll compose my life when the dust settles. I need a kinder, gentler life.

With this illness, my priorities became crystal clear. I don't want to lose that clarity even if the death threat is gone. Any guilt I used to feel about doing what I want to do instead of what I "should" do has vanished; I've paid my dues many times over. I want to spend more time with David and the kids, and I don't want to waste time and energy on stuff that is less meaningful. I hope I can keep my eye on the ball.

Love
Laura

From: Junior Faculty Council (JFC)
Sent: Tuesday, June 19, 2007 2:07 PM
To: Faculty
Subject: 2007 Award for Excellence in Mentoring

1st Annual Memorial Hospital Award for Excellence in Mentoring

This award was established to recognize outstanding commitment to mentoring and will be given annually to a Memorial Hospital faculty member nominated and selected by the Junior Faculty. We received many outstanding nominations and congratulate all who were nominated.

This year's recipient is:
Laura Liberman, M.D.
Attending Radiologist, Breast Imaging
Director, Breast Imaging Research Programs
Director, Program for Women Faculty Affairs
Memorial Sloan-Kettering Cancer Center
Member, Memorial Hospital
Professor of Radiology
Weill Medical College of Cornell University

Congratulations, Laura! Thanks to all the Junior Faculty who shared their experiences.

JFC

From: Laura
Sent: Thursday, June 21, 2007 5:46 PM
To: Jennifer
Subject: Anniversary presents

Dearest Jen,

Thanks for your thoughtful anniversary gifts. The books are wonderful, and I didn't own any of them! I brought them with me to the hospital, but my mom finished writing her autobiography and sent me the manuscript, so I read that instead. It's called *My Life into Art*, and is about her development as an artist. My mom grew up in Israel and her brother and first boyfriend were killed in Israeli wars; her father died young of a heart attack. She has had too much loss in her life. I knew some of the stories but didn't know all the details. I think I understand her better. Did I tell you that she's been emailing me a Blue Mountain card every day since I told her that I have cancer? It makes me smile when I click on the link and the background music starts blaring out of the computer.

Emma is packing to go to sleepaway camp—she leaves June 30, a week from Saturday. I miss her so much when she's away. But she loves camp, and six weeks will go by pretty fast. Both kids have survived their exams and they are finally free. By the end, we were all exhausted. We may have limped to the finish line, but we got there.

The Junior Faculty at my hospital started an award for Mentor of the Year. There were 15 doctors and/or scientists nominated, and I won! They announced it at a seminar on Tuesday. I was so touched that I was actually speechless, which (as you know) is not my natural state. They gave me a plaque

I SIGNED AS THE DOCTOR

that says Mentor of the Year with my name. They forgot to engrave the year, and they wanted me to give them the plaque back so they could put the year on it, but I like it better this way—now every year I can look at it and think I'm still the Mentor of the Year.

David and I went out to hear music last night at the Blue Note, a jazz club—McCoy Tyner on piano, his trio, and Toots Thielmanns playing jazz harmonica. Toots is about 88 and hasn't been healthy, but he sure can play. It's amazing to hear those sounds coming out of a harmonica. I spent too many years being in the office for too many hours a day. I want to spend more time with my family now, and take walks by the river, and listen to music, and read, and write.

I have more I'd tell you but there is a reception for medical students who are participating in a summer NIH program and I want to do my part to welcome them. I'm wearing a special hat for the occasion called the Ruby, which has a beige crown, medium brim, and off-white silk organza roses and bows.

Please keep in touch. I love to hear from you.

Love always
Laura

_____

From: Laura
Sent: Saturday, June 23, 2007 6:57 PM
To: Jennifer
Subject: Grace

Hi Jen. Today I went to visit a friend of mine in the hospital. Her name is Grace, and she works in the Radiology Department at Memorial, scheduling general radiology exams. I've known her for years. She's a quiet person in her 40s, very thoughtful and spiritual.

I found out that a couple of weeks ago, she showed up for work as usual around 7 am, and in the middle of taking a phone call she collapsed and became unresponsive. It looked like she was having some disaster in her brain. They took her to New York Hospital right across the street (we're connected by a tunnel), where she was immediately admitted. They did a bunch of tests, and apparently she had a stroke. She's been in the Neuro Intensive Care Unit ten days now.

When I was strolling this morning, after I walked south on the boardwalk, I went down a flight of stairs and kept walking south until I got to the exit at 71st Street, and then I went over a little walking bridge to get back to the street. The entrance to New York Hospital is on 70th Street between York and the River. I showed the people at the NYH information desk my Memorial ID, and was given permission to go up to the Neuro ICU. When I got to the ICU, I was surprised at how young all the doctors looked, and then I remembered that it's July, the time of year when the experienced doctors-in-training leave and new ones start.

I found Grace. She was in her own "room," really more a cubicle with a curtain separating it from the other cubicles. She was lying in bed. Her entire body was massively swollen, probably due to having received lots of IV fluid to stabilize her when she was admitted. She had tubes and lines everywhere—a nasogastric tube going through her nose into her stomach, an intravenous line in each arm to deliver fluids and medications, an arterial line in her wrist to check the oxygenation of her blood, and a catheter in her bladder to collect her urine. She couldn't move her body on the left side.

I leaned over so that I was in her field of view. She couldn't speak, but her eyes seemed to smile with recognition. One of the new young doctors came in, accompanied by an older doctor—the new intern, supervised by his more experienced resident. They said they were going to have to put another tube in her called a Swan Ganz catheter (also known as a "Swan") that they insert into a vein in the neck and thread into the heart to monitor the pressures at different levels in the circulation. They asked me to leave but I told them that I've been a doctor at Memorial for 17 years and that I have done and watched countless procedures. They let me stay.

I tried to imagine what it felt like to be Grace at that moment. She could see what was going on around her and recognize people but was unable to talk, and nobody explained what they were doing and why. I took her right hand, which she was still able to move, and softly told her what had happened. "You had a stroke, Grace," I said. "You're at New York Hospital in the Intensive Care Unit, and you've been here for 10 days. They have all these tubes in to give you nutrition and medicine. You can't move your left side because of the stroke. Often there are things you can't do right after a stroke, because the stroke damages brain cells. After you're stable, you're going to have rehabilitation and physical therapy so that you get back as much as possible."

She seemed to nod with her eyes, although she couldn't move her head.

The intern started to clean her skin and put a sterile drape over her neck in preparation for the Swan. I could feel her fear. I explained, "Now they're putting in another tube so they can monitor the pressures in your heart." I had my iPod, which I always bring when I take my walks. I put one of the earpieces in her ear and played a song from the musical Spring Awakening called "I Believe." It sounds like a gospel song, and the lyrics keep repeating, "I believe there is love in heaven. I believe all will be forgiven." When the song ended, I just played it again, a continuous loop of faith.

Grace's right hand, which had been tense in mine, relaxed. By the time the intern had finished inserting the Swan and putting the final stitches into the skin, Grace's breathing was rhythmic and steady, and I saw that she was asleep. She must have been exhausted. I let go of her hand, kissed her on the cheek, whispered "God bless you," and left. My friend Hilda has suggested to me and other friends of Grace that together we should get Grace her own iPod, which is a wonderful idea. Grace has a daughter who is computer-savvy and can put music on it for her. I thought about Grace and the iPod as I walked north along the East River, up the stairs, on the boardwalk, and then home.

You know how sometimes when someone is sick, you want to comfort them, but you don't how to help? That's how I felt when my father had his worst stroke, but it wasn't the case today. When I saw Grace, I was certain about what to do and how to do it. Cancer has given me that.

Love
Laura

From: Laura
Sent: Sunday, June 24, 2007 8:54 PM
To: Jennifer
Subject: Tea with Emma

Hi Jen. Today Emma and I went out for tea. We've had a tradition of going out for tea together for several years now. A few years ago, we got a book called *The New York Book of Tea*, which lists places in New York City "to have tea and buy teaware." We looked in the book, marked the places that interested us, and systematically explored them. Emma especially loves Earl Grey tea, and we're both fond of those tiny tea sandwiches, especially the ones with cucumber and watercress. And going to tea gives us a chance to talk.

We've tried a lot of tea places together. The Lobby Lounge at the Stanhope Hotel has Limoges china, with delicate designs of birds and flowers. The Mayfair Regent has a fruit snack with mixed berries. And the Gallery at the Carlyle, probably our favorite, has soft lighting and plush couches, and they serve "high tea" on a large silver multi-level platter, with three tiers: tiny sandwiches on the bottom, scones in the middle, and desserts on top. Next to the tea place inside the Carlyle is Bemelmans bar, which features walls hand-painted by the guy who illustrated the Madeleine books.

Today we went to the Gallery at the Carlyle. I wore a hat called the Erica, which has a square forest green crown, medium up-tilting brim, and a trim of lavender silk binding and roses. We asked for the high tea, with two orders of tiny tea sandwiches and no desserts. We tried a new kind of lemon tea which was tart and fragrant. We brought the Sunday paper and looked at the theater section to see what other musicals are in town. I want to get us tickets for some shows that we can see together after Emma gets back from camp. If we have the tickets, maybe the time she's away will go by faster.

Love
Laura

Chapter 13
Chemo Ends

Hope.

From: Laura
Sent: Saturday, June 30, 2007 2:15 PM
To: Jennifer
Subject: Emma went to camp

Hi Jen. Today we took Emma to the bus to go to her sleepaway camp, which is called Mountainview in upstate New York. When she was younger, and went to day camp, they had a one-week optional trip to Mountainview, and she loved it. She started going there the summer after that; this will be her fourth summer there.

The bus leaves from 5th Avenue on the Upper East Side. Because they're only allowed to bring two small bags on the bus, we have to ship most of her stuff in advance. It's funny—there's a weekend in early June where every kid in the building seems to be sending their bags to camp—the lobby is littered with duffel bags, suitcases, and trunks, ready for pick-up by the various camp trucking services. So we had sent most of Emma's things already, but there were still a few items she packed at the last minute.

Dropping her off is always bittersweet. She loves her camp friends and has always had a terrific time at camp, but it's hard to say goodbye, especially since they don't allow the kids to have cell phones or Internet access. We can email her letters, and the camp prints them out and delivers them to the kids during "mail time," which is every day after lunch. We're allowed two phone calls and one visit.

We always have to get to the bus about an hour early, to help her load up her luggage and to touch base with her counselors. It's great to see how happy Emma is to reunite with her friends, and how delighted they are to see her. After the luggage is loaded and the kids take their seats, everybody waves and the bus takes off. I'll write to her. And by the time she gets home, my chemo will be done.

Love
Laura

From: Laura
Sent: Sunday, July 1 2007 10:00 AM
To: Emma
Subject: Camp

Dearest Emma,

It's Sunday morning at 9:30 am. I can't believe you've only been gone one day! It feels like longer. We got the "safe arrival" phone call from camp late yesterday afternoon, so I know you're OK. Did you have your swim test? If so, what was the effect of the chlorine on your beautiful washed and blown-dry hair?

The rest of the day after dropping you off was uneventful. Dad took me home and then he went to work. I went out to drop off clothes at the dry cleaners and then to the Vinegar Factory to get some fruit—we were out of plums. I came home and tried to nap, but couldn't. After a couple of hours, Dad came home and fell asleep on the couch in the living room, reading. Nate went out and I went up to the pool around 5 pm. I swam laps for 40 minutes and then came downstairs. Dad had already woken up. I took a shower and got dressed for dinner—the sleeveless black dress with a silver sparkly jacket from Eileen Fisher that I haven't worn yet, with my favorite hat (the Butterfly—mauve crown with muted gold silk bow). We took a cab and picked up the Sterns to go out to dinner.

The restaurant we went to was one we'd been to before, called Knickerbockers. The food was delicious. I had sole and Dad had a T-bone steak, and they had the best onion rings I had ever tasted. Dad, John, and Hannah shared a chocolate souffle for dessert. Hannah was wearing the elegant gold jacket that was part of the suit she wore at Sarah's graduation, with jeans. It was a great combination. We had fun with them. Sarah already left for camp; Lisa is still around, but will be going to softball camp for a week and then to be a counselor at her old camp for about a month. After dinner, a trio played jazz; the pianist is someone John and Hannah know, who played at both girls' Bat Mitzvahs.

I'm going to take it easy today. I'll take a walk and go to the pool to cool off. I'll read in the air conditioning, and then maybe do one of my favorite things — napping!

I love you very much, Emma. I can't wait to hear about camp, your bunkmates, your counselors, and what you're doing. Where is your bed? Did you set it up with the soft blanket and pillow?

Much love
Sun Moon Stars
Mom

From: Laura
Sent: Tuesday, July 3, 2007 6:11 am
To: Emma
Subject: This and that

Dearest Emma,

On Sunday, I hung around most of the day, working on the computer and reading the paper. Then in the afternoon I went for a walk by the river, and then a swim. Since Sunday was July 1, the pool is now open until 8 every night, and 9 on Wednesdays. When I came back to the apartment, Dad had been giving Nate a cooking lesson. They covered some important ground—meat and potatoes. Dad showed Nate how to make a steak, which came out delicious, but Nate said really Dad made it. The good news is, no matter what becomes of Nate's cooking skills, he will always be able to order out.

Yesterday was a good day at work. It was quiet—when July 4 falls on Wednesday, some people take off Monday & Tuesday, and others take off Thursday & Friday, so it ends up being quiet for the whole week. I'm off tomorrow for the 4th of July. We'll probably sleep late and go to the pool.

I hope you're having a fantastic time at camp. I can't wait to hear the stories. I love you always.

Love
Sun Moon Stars
Mom

From: Laura
Sent: Wednesday, July 4, 2007 11:02 AM
To: Emma
Subject: 4th of July

Dearest Emma,

Happy 4th of July!

Today looks light for all of us. No work, and Nate is still sleeping. Dad is writing to you now on his laptop. We may go see the Michael Moore movie "Sicko" later. They had a sign up in the elevator for the fireworks on the roof, which was odd because with the new building next door you can't really see the fireworks anymore. It's gray today but not raining yet, so I may swim.

Emma, I only have 22 days (less than a month!) left before July 26, which is the date of my last chemo. I am so excited—I want to buy a big bunch of pink balloons and release them when it's all finished.

Have a wonderful day today and every day at camp.

Love always
Sun Moon Stars
Mom

From: Laura
Sent: Sunday, July 8, 2007 6:14 AM
To: Emma
Subject: New Jersey

Dearest Emma,

    Today is Sunday. The boys are still sleeping, but I'm awake.

.   Yesterday I had fun! My friend Cindy invited me and two friends of ours who we work with to her house in New Jersey. We met at 10:30 am at the Time Warner Building, and drove to New Jersey. We had each brought flowers. There was almost no traffic, so it only took about 20 minutes to drive there.

    The house, which is in Fort Lee, NJ, has three floors. The lowest floor is this huge beautiful open common space, with a kitchen that has tiles like ours, and a family room that has a dining area. Then, on the second floor, there's a sitting room, formal dining room, and 2nd kitchen. The third floor has three bedrooms and an office. There is a front yard and a gorgeous back area with an in-ground pool, table and chairs, and a fabulous garden, and it's all surrounded by tall trees, so it was nice and cool and shady even though it was hot outside. The house is nicer than any place we've ever rented in Hilton Head! I asked Cindy if we could spend our vacations at her house. She laughed.

    They had made such delicious food. Cindy's significant other, Juan, made the most spectacular guacamole I have ever tasted, right in front of us. He explained what he was doing as he went along. It reminded me of the TV show where all these chefs audition to see who gets his/her own Food Network Show—Juan would have won, hands down! They also grilled chicken and made this delicious salad with orzo and vegetables. I felt like we were eating all day!

    After lunch, we all jumped in the pool. We floated around and talked. That's where I was when you called—I am so sorry that I missed your call! But I hear from Dad and Nate that you're doing great. After 5 we came back to the city.

My friend Hilda gave me a terrific DVD called Mad Hot Ballroom, which is a documentary about a bunch of New York City public high school kids who learned ballroom dancing and participated in a dance competition. Dad and I watched it last night after I got home. You would love it—when you get home, we'll watch it together.

I'm getting admitted to the hospital on Thursday of next week, which will hopefully be my last admission, and should be home by Monday. Dad will come to Visitors' Day this Saturday without me because I'll still be in the hospital. We got permission for both of us to come back to visit you at camp on Sunday 7/22.

How'd you get to be so beautiful?

Love
Sun Moon Stars
Mom

From: Laura
Sent: Thursday, July 12, 2007 3:38 PM
To: Emma
Subject: Last admission

Dearest Emma,

I just got to the hospital for my last admission! I have the same room that I had the first time I was admitted. When I logged onto AOL, your login came up—you must have been the last one to use it. This is the room that has the bulletin board where you arranged the pins to spell your name, remember? The pins are still there, and they still say "Emma." I love those signs of you; they make me feel like you're here with me. I'm getting a late start on chemo today, so I'll probably go home Monday.

It's been incredibly hot for the last two days. Tuesday in particular was unbelievable. They had a picnic for lunch at my work but it was too hot for me to go! Today is a little cooler (finally). It rained last night, and I think that broke the heat.

This morning I took my walk on the boardwalk, and I went to the Vinegar Factory to get fruit for this admission. I got plums and cherries and nectarines and pluots and grapes. That should do for a few days. Dad will bring them when he brings my clothes later. And, of course, frozen yogurt.

There is a pile of bags in the hall of the stuff Dad is going to bring you to camp on Visitors' Day this Saturday. You guys will have a wonderful time. I love you so much.

Much love
Sun Moon Stars
Mom

From: Laura
Sent: Thursday, July 12, 2007 2:41 PM
To: Cindy
Subject: Balloons

Hi Cindy. Can you remind me where you got the beautiful bouquet of pink balloons that you gave me for my birthday? I want to order some. Thanks!

Love
Laura

From: Laura
Sent: Sunday, July 15, 2007 7:40 AM
To: Emma
Subject: Home today?

Dearest Emma,

It's Sunday morning. I've been up since 5:30. I walked laps around the nursing station for an hour. They checked my pulse, temperature, and blood pressure, and they sent some blood tests to the lab. The one I care about the most is the methotrexate level—if it's under 50, I get to go home today. I can't believe that this may be my last admission—#5 of 5 admissions, and chemo #15 out of 16.

Q came to visit yesterday. She brought me the book *On Chesil Beach* by Ian McEwan, and showed me some new digital photos of Nick and Ben. After Q left, Dad came. It was a little after 4. He said he had a wonderful time visiting you at camp. We watched a rerun of Monk on the hospital TV and took a nap together. Nate went out with his friends and I didn't see him yesterday.

I finished the fabulous book I was reading: *Eat, Pray, Love* by Elizabeth Gilbert. It's about a woman who goes through a bitter divorce and depression and then takes a three-part trip, to Italy (to discover the pleasures of the body—"eat"), India (to discover spiritual pleasures—"pray"), and Indonesia (to find the balance between the two—"love"). I loved it! When she goes to Italy, she describes all the delicious food she eats. She would get to a town and ask, "Where do you get the best food in this town?" And when she went to a restaurant, she would say, "Don't bring me the menu—just bring me the best meal you can cook." Her food descriptions make your mouth water. Definitely something you want to read near a stocked refrigerator or take-out menus. The story is genuine and the writing riveting.

I've just got 11 days left, Emma. And I'll see you at camp a week from today, in seven days. I love you so much.

Love
Sun Moon Stars
Mom

From: Laura
Sent: Saturday, July 21, 2007 5:58 AM
To: Emma
Subject: Tomorrow

Dearest Emma,

It's Saturday morning at almost 6 am, and I'm writing to you on my laptop. The boys are still asleep. It looks like another beautiful day. I have no plans for the day except resting.

Emma, I have five more days left until I'm done with chemo! And the countdown continues. I can't wait until it's over. I also can't wait until I see you tomorrow—Dad and I are taking you out to a delicious lunch! And I'm going to give you a great big hug. I love you very much.

Much love
Sun Moon Stars
Mom

From: Laura
Sent: Thursday, July 26, 2007 9:12 PM
To: Emma
Subject: Finale

Dearest Emma,
  I'm DONE WITH CHEMO!!!!!!!!!!!!!!!!!!!!!!!!!!!!!!!!!!
The pre-celebration started yesterday. I ordered 2 dozen
rainbow-colored balloons in various shapes (stars, hearts, etc.)
and 1 dozen pink balloons, all made of Mylar instead of latex
(because some people have allergies to latex) to be delivered to
the hospital yesterday afternoon. I ordered them from the
Balloon Salloon, which is where my work friends had ordered
the balloons we got for my birthday just as I was beginning
chemo. Great place—Tiffany, the balloon expert, was very
helpful, and when you're on hold you get to listen to a great
song that goes "Let's go sail away in my beautiful balloon,"
which I have loved since I was a kid.
  For an extra 50 cents per balloon, you can get a special
treatment that makes the balloons stay on the ceiling for a week
instead of a day. When I told them I'm getting the balloons to
celebrate the end of chemo, Tiffany said that they would throw
in the treatment for free (that may be the last time I get to "play
the cancer card!"). So yesterday these 3 dozen balloons were
delivered to the Women's Office. I brought the 2 dozen
rainbow-colored balloons in various shapes to Athena, our
informal group for women faculty, to celebrate the last night
before chemo.
  Bringing the balloons to the meeting was harder than I
had predicted. Have you ever tried to get through a revolving
door with two dozen helium-filled balloons? Let me tell you
right now, it doesn't work. Luckily we found an alternative,
non-revolving door. Then when we got to the Faculty Club,

where Athena is held, we released the balloons. Unfortunately, when we did it, we were standing in a part of the room with a particularly high ceiling, and the balloons all flew way up to the ceiling, where we couldn't retrieve them. The tallest woman among us, Ann, stood on a chair with tongs and managed to retrieve several balloons, and we took them to a part of the room with lower ceilings, so we could reach them.

The meeting was great. We celebrated three women's promotions. One of the women brought her mom, her two daughters, and the people who work with her in the office. We gave them each a bouquet of flowers. I told them I was celebrating the end of chemo. It was warm and supportive and wonderful. I got a lot of hugs. When I came home, Dad and Nate were here. Dad had ordered me some delicious fruit from Harry & David—cherries, plums, and peaches, which are my favorite.

Today was the last day of chemo. I woke up around 6, but went back to sleep until 7. I showered and got dressed (Caribbean skirt, brown silk sleeveless Eileen Fisher tank, Monk hat) and went to check in at chemo. Then two hours in my office while they mixed the chemo. I got my favorite room, with windows, and had two neighbors—a woman named Georgina and a woman named Bella. My nurse was Beth. The chemo went in fine—no problems. At 1:06 pm, I heard the three beeps of the pump that indicated that my Rituximab was in— the last of the chemo! They had to give me a little more IV fluid, and they disconnected me at 1:36 pm.

I gave balloons to Cindy, Beth, my neighbors in the chemo suite, the nurses and patients in the other chemo suite, the people at the front desk, Phil, and a few others. And then I came home.

I had ordered an additional 50 helium balloons (latex— we're not allergic to latex at home and they're cheaper), in all different shades of pink, to be delivered to the apartment. When I got home, Dad, Nate, and the balloons were here. We released the balloons in the apartment, and they flew to the ceiling of the living room, with their long strings hanging down—just like at the beginning of chemo. I like the symmetry, starting and ending with the same celebration. We're going to do what we did before—liberate the balloons that lose helium from the terrace into the sky. Today one balloon had no string, so we liberated it—and off it went, and it was gone—and hopefully my cancer is gone too.

I'll have post-chemo tests in a month. If the tests are good, I get maintained on a medicine called Rituximab, which I'll probably get once every two months intravenously as an outpatient. If the tests are bad, I get a bone marrow transplant. The tests in the middle of chemo were good, and hopefully these will be too.

I'm going to take it easy for a few days. Next weekend we'll start packing for Nate's trip to Spain. And the three of us will spend a long weekend in Maine before you get home.

Emma, it was so wonderful to see you this past Sunday and to hear about camp. I loved our lunch and trip to the mall—I'm excited about doing more serious shopping with you when you get home! And don't worry, I'll be off prednisone by then, so you don't have to worry that when I find shoes I like, that I will buy them in every color.

Much Love Always
Sun Moon Stars
And Everything Beautiful in the Universe
Mom

From: Laura
Sent: Thursday, July 26, 2007 11:14 PM
To: Jennifer
Subject: Done with chemo!

Dearest Jen,

I know how busy you are with the baby, but this is just a quick note to share with you—today was my last day of chemo! The post-chemo work-up (CT, MRI, bone marrow) is in a month, and will determine the next steps.

Kiss the kids for me, and let's talk soon. You call me—I don't want to violate the golden rule, Never Awaken a Sleeping Baby.

Love
Laura

From: Laura
Sent: Friday, July 27, 2007 1:28 PM
To: Cindy
Subject: RE: You're gonna make it after all!

Cindy—I'm singing along! I was so thrilled you joined me in chemo to release the balloons. It was so fitting for you to be there. You were my guardian angel through the worst of the chemo, so I'm glad you could be there for the best!

Today when I took my walk I tied a pink balloon to my fanny pack (on the side; otherwise if I tied it in the back it would look like I have a large pink tail). I was curious to see how people on the boardwalk would respond. One guy with sunglasses who was running gave me a thumbs up, and I gave him a thumbs up in return; everyone else ignored it. Typical New Yorkers. I could walk down the boardwalk on fire and nobody would pay attention. Got to love this town.

Love
Laura

From: Laura
Sent: Tuesday, July 31, 2007 4:48 AM
To: Jennifer
Subject: The Prednisone Diaries: Finale

Dearest Jen,
    Today is my last day of prednisone! I had my final R-CHOP on Thursday, with 5 days of oral prednisone afterwards (Friday, Saturday, Sunday, Monday, Tuesday). Today's Tuesday, so that's it— "The Prednisone Diaries" finale!
    Update on the 50 helium-filled pink balloons I had delivered to my apartment at the end of chemo—David, Nate and I placed bets on how long the last balloon would be up on the ceiling. I guessed August 2, but they're almost all down now (mine might still be the closest bet—Nate and David picked August 3 and 4, respectively). Today Nate and I liberated some balloons off the terrace, and they soared into the sky.
    It ain't over, Jen—the post-chemo work-up will be late August/early September. Rituximab or a bone marrow transplant. Come on, Rituximab!

Love
Laura

From: Laura
Sent: Tuesday, July 31, 2007 6:00 PM
To: Emma
Subject: To Emma in Washington DC

Dearest Emma,

It's Tuesday night. Are you done or almost done with your Washington trip? Did you have a good time?

Yesterday I worked a regular day, but today was lighter. I had to go to a doctor's appointment this morning for some blood tests and a shot (all of which were fine) and then I gave a noon seminar to new faculty members at my hospital on how to get promoted.

After the seminar was done I got in a cab to go home and called Dad—and he was already at home. Can you imagine? We were both home by 2:00 in the afternoon! Carmen had already left for the day and Nate was out. We went up to the pool for a swim, read a little, and came downstairs, made a big salad with grilled chicken, and watched a jazz video on DVD— Art Blakey and the Jazz Messengers playing a bunch of songs including one that was really great called "Moanin'."

Now I have something else to count down. It's July 31, and on August 10 you're done with camp. Ten more days until my beautiful Emma comes home. I love you so much, Emma.

Much love
Sun Moon Stars
Mom

From: Laura
Sent: Wednesday, August 1, 2007 4:31 AM
To: Jennifer
Subject: Getting together

Hi Jen. I'm so excited that you're making a day trip to New York in a couple of weeks. August 18 is perfect! Can you come to my house for lunch, and I'll make gazpacho and get fresh bread? We can eat on the terrace if it's not too hot, and otherwise we can eat inside in the air conditioning. Let's talk and make a definite plan.

David, Nate and I are going to Maine for a long weekend while Emma is still in camp. I used to go to camp in Maine when I was a kid and remember the rough wild beauty of the place. It will be great to relax and breathe. Emma gets home on August 10, and then Nate goes to Spain the next day.

Love
Laura

From: Laura
Sent: Friday, August 31, 2007 10:07 AM
To: Jennifer
Subject: Post-treatment work-up

Hi Jen. It was so wonderful to see you when you came to New York and to meet Benjamin! I'm glad you got to see Emma too. Nate's having a terrific time in Spain, and will be home soon. David and I are enjoying the last days of summer.

This week I had my post-treatment work-up and the CT, MRI, and repeat bone marrow biopsies were negative! They said "NO EVIDENCE OF LYMPHOMA" three times. No bone marrow transplant—I'm thrilled! I'll get maintenance Rituximab for at least six months, and then they'll repeat the tests to confirm that I'm still in remission. The minute I found out, I called David at work, Nate in Spain, and Emma at home from my cell phone to tell them the good news. As I took my celebratory walk home on the boardwalk, I couldn't help dancing as Marvin Gaye and Tammi Terrell sang, "Ain't No Mountain High Enough."

When I got home, I told Emma that I hope to be around to embarrass her for years to come. She said to me, "Mom, could you be around, but NOT embarrass me?" And I said, "Oh, no, honey, that's not possible. Moms have been embarrassing their teenage daughters since the dawn of time. We can't break with tradition."

Love
Laura

Chapter 14
How to Cope with Cancer: Lists

From: Laura
Sent: Tuesday, September 04, 2007 11:07 AM
To: Jennifer
Subject: Lists

Hi Jen. Based on my experience as both a cancer doctor and a cancer patient, I've written lists of suggestions about how to cope with cancer. For individuals dealing with cancer and for their loved ones, I have a general list of 18 items—in Hebrew, the symbol for 18 is "Chai," which means life. I also give a list of reading material, music, and other activities that may help those with cancer. In addition, I provide a list of suggestions for doctors caring for individuals with cancer. The lists follow.

List 1: For Those with Cancer & Their Loved Ones

1. Reach out to your friends.
2. It's OK to cry, but do so ≤20 minutes/day.
3. Ask for what you need. Be your own advocate.
4. Cancer is the best excuse you'll ever have—use it! "Play the cancer card."
5. Get your priorities straight.
6. Keep your sense of humor.
7. Find silver linings. Don't look at this as losing your hair, but rather as an opportunity to get new hats!
8. Get doctors you trust and listen to their advice.

9. Be sensitive to your family. Tell them that it's OK to talk about it. It can be harder on them than on you.
10. Get in shape, physically and mentally. Save your energy for the fight. Don't sweat the small stuff or anticipate too much in advance. Take it "bird by bird."
11. Use your experience to help others.
12. Bring your own anesthesia, like ethyl chloride spray and Emla cream. Ask your doctor for a prescription. If you need lots of IV chemo, strongly consider getting a port (catheter) before treatment—it will spare you multiple needle sticks.
13. Go iPod!! Have your partner, friends, family, and/or kids put songs on it. Listen during chemo. Read books. Curl up with family & friends, and watch DVDs (try Monk—it's great and each episode lasts an hour).
14. Discover your inner Zen. You will have to wait a lot. Pretend each doctor's visit is a trip to the airport.
15. Savor celebrations. It's not all about the cancer!
16. Ask people to pray for you. Have all denominations covered. Befriend a Buddhist.
17. Write about it.
18. Hope.

List 2: Suggested Reading

BOOKS: CANCER OR ILLNESS-RELATED

Bauby JD. *The Diving Bell and the Butterfly: A Memoir of Life in Death.* New York, NY: Vintage Books, Random House, Inc.; 1998

Bolte-Taylor, J. *My Stroke of Insight: A Brain Scientist's Personal Journey.* New York, NY: Viking Press; 1998 (Especially helpful are Chapter 20, Tending the Garden, and Appendix B, Forty Things I Needed the Most.)

Genova, L. *Still Alice.* New York, NY: Pocket Books, Simon & Schuster, Inc.; 2009

Gould SJ. *Full House: The Spread of Excellence from Plato to Darwin.* New York, NY: Three Rivers Press; 1996 (especially Chapter 4, Case One: A Personal Story, Where any measure of central tendency acts as a harmful abstraction, and variation stands out as the only meaningful reality, pp 45-56; note Figure 7 on page 55)

Holland J and Lewis, S. *The Human Side of Cancer: Living with Hope, Coping with Uncertainty.* New York, NY: HarperCollins Publishers; 2000

Pausch R with Zaslow G. *The Last Lecture.* New York, NY: Hyperion Books; 2008 ("We cannot change the cards we're dealt, just how we play the hand.") Also, see his amazing YouTube video at http://www.youtube.com/watch?v+jv_Mqcs=xdo

BOOKS: OTHER

Cunningham M. *The Hours*. New York, NY: Picador; 2000

Daniell E. *Every Other Thursday: Stories and Strategies from Successful Women Scientists*. New Haven, CT: Yale University Press; 2008

Gilbert E. *Eat, Pray, Love: One Woman's Search for Everything Across Italy, India, and Indonesia*. New York, NY: Penguin Books; 2007

Kellaway L and Lukes M. *Who Moved My Blackberry?* New York, NY: Hyperion; 2006

Lamott A. *Bird by Bird: Some Instructions on Writing and Life*. New York, NY: Anchor Books, Random House; 1995

Niles B. *New York's 50 Best Places to Take Tea.* New York, NY: Universe Publishing; 2008 (If you're not a New Yorker, get a similar book for your home town, and *go!*)

Obama B. *The Audacity of Hope*: Thoughts on Reclaiming the American Dream. New York, NY: Crown Publishers, Random House; 2006

Patchett A. *Bel Canto*. New York, NY: HarperCollins; 2001

Quindlen A. *A Short Guide to a Happy Life*. New York, NY: Random House; 2000

SHORT STORIES

Carver R. *Where I'm Calling From*. New York, NY: Vintage Contemporaries; 1989 (or anything else by him)

Hemingway E. *The Complete Short Stories of Ernest Hemingway*. New York, NY: Scribner Paperback Fiction, Simon & Schuster; 1998 (or anything else by him)

Klass P. *Love and Modern Medicine*. New York, NY: Houghton Mifflin; 2001 (or anything else by her)

Lahiri, Jhumpa. *Unaccustomed Earth*. New York, NY: Alfred A. Knopf; 2008 (or anything else by her)

PLAYS

Edson M. *Wit*. New York, NY: Dramatists Play Service; 1999

Wasserstein W. *Third*. New York, NY: Dramatists Play Service (unpublished manuscript)

POETRY

Carver R. *All of Us: The Collected Poems*. New York, NY: Vintage; 2000

Dickinson E. *The Poems of Emily Dickinson: Reading Edition*. Belknap Press; 2005

List 3: Suggested Music, Listening, & Viewing

POPULAR

The Beach Boys Greatest Hits
The Beatles
George Benson
Joe Cocker, With a Little Help From My Friends
Sam Cooke, Portrait of a Legend
Feeling Groovy (Patrick and Eugene)
Aretha Franklin
Marvin Gaye, The Love Songs (& Ain't No Mountain High
    Enough)
Al Green (Greatest Hits)
The Jackson 5, I'll Be There
Norah Jones, Come Away With Me (or anything else she sings)
Ben E. King, Stand By Me
Carole King: Tapestry, Music, Rhymes & Reasons
Bette Midler: The Divine Miss M
Moon River
Diana Ross and the Supremes
Sade, Stronger than Pride
Frank Sinatra
Buffalo Springfield, For What It's Worth
James Taylor (Best of James Taylor)
Tears for Fears, Shout
The Temptations (My Girl, The Way You Do The Things
    You Do, anything else)
Three Dog Night (especially One, Eli's Coming, Joy to the
    World)
Stevie Wonder, At the Close of a Century

CLASSICAL

Bach (anything he wrote)
Bach: Hilary Hahn plays Bach
Bach: Piano Concertos, Partitas, Preludes and Fugues, 2- and
   3-part Inventions, Goldberg Variations, played by Glenn
   Gould
Bach Six Suites for Unaccompanied Cello, played by Yo-Yo
   Ma (or anything else played by him)
Beethoven Symphonies (eg #7 2nd movement & #9)
Beethoven piano sonatas, piano concertos
Brahms Sonatas for Cello and Piano, played by Yo-Yo Ma &
   Emanuel Ax
Brahms Sonatas for Clarinet and Piano, Clarinet Trio
Chopin Nocturnes
Elgar Cello Concerto by Jacqueline Du Pre (or anything else
   played by her)
Mozart Piano Concertos, played by Murray Perahia
Mozart Piano Sonatas, Sonatas for 1 Piano 4 Hands, Sonatas
   for 2 Pianos
Mozart Violin Sonatas, played by Hilary Hahn
Poulenc Clarinet Sonata, Flute Sonata
Schubert Impromptus, Fantastia in F Minor for two pianos,
   Trout Quintet, Unfinished Symphony
Schumann Kreisleriana, Fantasiestucke
Schumann: Music & the Mind, Vol I (DVD), The Life &
   Works of Robert Schumann, by Dr. Richard Kogan

JAZZ

Louis Armstrong:
 Louis Armstrong Meets Oscar Peterson, Louis Armstrong
 & Ella Fitzgerald
Chet Baker
Joanne Brackeen
Dee Dee Bridgewater
Betty Carter
Ray Charles (especially Georgia on My Mind)
John Coltrane (especially My Favorite Things, My One &
 Only Love)
Eddie Daniels: To Bird With Love
Miles Davis, Kind of Blue
Eliane Elias, Something for You (sings and plays Bill Evans)
Bill Evans; Bill Evans & Jim Hall
Ella Fitzgerald
Getz/Gilberto (especially The Girl From Ipanema,
 Corcovado)
Dexter Gordon
Jim Hall, Concierto
Herbie Hancock, Speak Like a Child
Keith Jarrett (At the Deer Head Inn or any trio)
Nino Josele (jazz guitar; especially playing the music of Bill
 Evans)
Jeremy Pelt
Houston Person (especially It Might As Well Be Spring)
Oscar Peterson
Toots Theilemans
Sarah Vaughan
Ben Webster; Ben Webster Meets Oscar Peterson
Joe Williams
Cassandra Wilson (Blue Skies, Standards)

MUSICAL THEATER

A Chorus Line
Company
Dreamgirls
Hairspray
In the Heights
Mo' Better Blues
Rent
Singin' in the Rain
Spring Awakening
Wicked

DVD/TV

The Colbert Report with Stephen Colbert
The Daily Show with Jon Stewart
Hitchcock movies
Monk
Project Runway
The Rachel Maddow Show
Sports Night
West Wing
Woody Allen movies

COMEDY

George Carlin

List 4: Advice to Doctors

1. The person you are treating is not just a "patient," but an individual, with a life, a brain, and a heart.
2. Listen to those you treat and their loved ones.
3. Give essential information. Be honest, and don't abolish hope.
4. Be kind and respectful. Let the people in your care keep their dignity.
5. Encourage those for whom you care to deal with each item as it arises, and not to anticipate several steps in advance. Understand that this is easier said than done.
6. Realize what you do and don't know. If you don't know something, learn it or ask someone who does.
7. Treat as you would want to be treated. The white coat doesn't make you immune. One day, you may be on the other side.
8. Relieve pain. Be generous with anesthesia.
9. Alleviate anxiety and fear. Cancer can be scary.
10. Cure us or put us into remission, if you can. If not, help each of us live what we perceive to be the best life possible.

I'd appreciate any edits.

Love
Laura

Afterword

Write about it.

From: Laura
Sent: Thursday, March 20, 2008 3:47 am
To: Jennifer
Subject: Looking back

Hi Jen. I haven't written you a middle-of-the-night email for a long time. So many stories to tell!

It's been a tough six months since I went into remission. I was exhausted and went into a depression that lasted for several months. While you're getting chemo, you're highly focused and the adrenaline is pumping. All of your energy is geared to fighting cancer, which has got to be one of the world's best enemies. There's no time or energy to reflect. The agenda is simple: survival. You hang on for dear life. Then the battle ends, and some people think that once the cancer is in remission, you're done, and you can go back to business as usual. They're wrong. Surviving cancer is like weathering Hurricane Katrina. After the storm has passed, it takes time to survey the damage and rebuild.

The post-chemo depression took me by surprise. It's hard to accept that your body isn't the same as it used to be. Before cancer, I had been highly energetic: Picture the Eveready Bunny ("it keeps going and going...") in the hospital, juggling multiple activities at once, and that was me. After chemo, I had to learn to live with fatigue and with a new cognitive style: I could no longer multi-task. I've since spoken to lots of cancer survivors, who tell me that diminished multitasking ability after chemo is fairly common. Changes in your body or persona can be experienced as a loss, and as with any loss, you may grieve. It helped to view the depression as a foggy beach, with the sun hidden behind it; I knew that somewhere in there the sun was shining, and that eventually I'd find it. I also used my hospital's survivorship program when I could, although sometimes it wasn't possible—for example, one night they had a lecture on "Coping with Fatigue after Cancer Treatment," but I was too tired to go!

The chemo part of my treatment is over, but I'm continuing on maintenance therapy for at least two years. Once every two months, I get an infusion of Rituximab, the monoclonal antibody against B lymphocytes that had been the R of the R-CHOP regimen that I received during chemo. I've kept the port in my chest, so they can give the Rituximab through that. Because the monoclonal antibody treatment compromises my immune system, I continue to take a slew of pills to prevent infection. The chemo put me into menopause, so I take hormone replacement—until I started taking it, I was constantly throwing open the windows on freezing cold days, and David would have to go put on a warm pair of socks.

A surgeon I know once told me that as a working mom, you juggle three things: (1) work, (2) family, and (3) taking care of yourself; at any given time, you get to focus on two out of three. Item (3) is especially challenging when you're dealing with ongoing treatment and the aftermath of chemo. To accommodate my body, I now work four days a week: two in the Women's Office (Mondays and Wednesdays) and two in Radiology (Tuesdays and Fridays). Friday is the day I see patients and do procedures. Thursday is my day off and it fills easily, with doctors' appointments, music, reading, tea with Q, and naps. I sleep for most of the weekend to recover from doing clinical work on Fridays.

Having cancer changes you in unexpected ways. I selectively use my experience to help patients. Sometimes if I tell a patient that she has cancer and she takes it hard, I tell her that I'm a cancer survivor and share with her the survival skills I learned, including finding your friends, asking for what you want, getting an iPod, and "playing the cancer card." I also give lots more anesthesia for procedures than I did before. It's odd how when I was first diagnosed, I felt like a doctor pretending to be a patient. Now, sometimes I feel like a patient pretending to be a doctor. The other day, I did a biopsy on a woman with a breast lump, and when I signed the consent, I signed as the patient!

Sometimes friends ask me how I stayed so calm during chemo—why didn't I "lose it" more often? (Funny, my super, Jesus, never asks me that.) The survival techniques I described in the lists I sent you helped a lot. In addition, cancer gave me something I hadn't ever given myself—a break. I'd always been an intense workaholic. Having cancer forced me to slow down and look around, and once I looked around, I liked what I saw. If I had to have cancer, I'm glad that it happened when both of my kids were still at home so I could spend time with them. I can't redo the past, but I can use my experience to attain a better balance in the rest of my life and to help others find balance in theirs. Now that's a real silver lining.

After I finished treatment, I spent several weeks cutting and pasting all of the emails I had written about my experience (mostly to you) into a Word document for the book I'd planned, but when I finally put it together, the book was 951 pages long. The idea of cutting that massive tome into a book of manageable size was daunting. The information was so raw and fresh that I didn't feel I could cut any of it—it was all too important—so I put it away for awhile. Now, six months later, I'm still exhausted but the fog of depression has lifted. I started thinking that I'd like to turn the book into a series of interconnected short stories, and that it would help me accomplish that if I met other writers off whom to bounce ideas.

Nate went online with me to look for writing classes. He found the Gotham Writers' Workshop, a funky New York group that has writing classes all over the city. I found a course that meets on Wednesday nights on the Upper East Side, about halfway between work and my house. I thought that would be perfect, especially since I'm in the Women's Office on Wednesdays so I shouldn't be as exhausted as after a day of biopsies. Also, I don't work on Thursdays, so if I'm inspired by the workshop on Wednesday night, I have the next day to write.

The class started in early March, and I love it. The teacher, Tania, got her Master's at Columbia, and will publish her first novel in the fall. There are 12 students, six women and six men. It's a diverse crowd, ranging from a kid Nate's age to a woman about to retire. Other students include a TV producer, a guy who writes advertising copy, a woman who teaches high school English, and a couple of people who work at Barnes & Noble. Another student is a woman in her twenties who takes pole dancing (when I told Emma the story, she rolled her eyes and said that pole dancing is popular; many celebrities do it for exercise. Who knew?). Most of the students want to write short stories but one man is working on a novel.

The best part of class is called "Booth." When it's your turn for booth, you have to give copies of 15-25 pages of original writing to all class participants. They take it home to read and give comments the next week. First, we go around the room and everyone gives a positive comment, and then we go around again and everyone gives an "improvement" comment. They needed a volunteer for week one, so I raised my hand. I had already decided to write about the hats Emma and I went to buy at the beginning of chemo. I thought I'd tell it from a third person point of view, lulling the reader with lush language describing the hats' colors and fabrics, and not revealing until the end that the woman is buying the hats because she is about to start chemo and lose her hair (and possibly her life). A surprise ending, like in "The Necklace" by Guy de Maupassant.

I went to the computer and opened my file marked "Book" and browsed through it for the first time since the fall. Amazing—what had looked so daunting to me before now seems absolutely manageable. It stands together as a book, and I'm going to write the book. When I look at the first draft carefully I see that sometimes I tell the same story several times to different people in different emails, so often I have multiple drafts of the same material. The redundancy makes it easier to trim and lets me choose the best elements of the story to combine into a cohesive whole. So when it's my turn for Booth, I bring in 15-25 pages of the book.

Since I've resumed writing, I've been waking up again from 3-5 am, now without the help of steroids. Maybe in writing the book I'm putting myself back into the frame of mind that I had during treatment, and maybe that will help me recreate the story. It will be a huge job. Even with the distance of six months, some of the stuff seems so precious that it's hard to cut, even if it doesn't serve the story. A writing teacher named Carol Winkelman once told me that when you're editing, sometimes you have to "slaughter your darlings," meaning cut something you wrote that's close to your heart. She suggested that rather than deleting, you simply cut and paste the section you're omitting into another file (I call mine "out-takes"). This technique makes it easier to edit because material isn't being destroyed, just relocated. Sometimes I think that my father wanted me to be a doctor and a writer—he used to tell me that Chekhov did both.

It seems appropriate that the end of my book is written about a year after treatment began. I'm spending more time with my family, and they're doing great. Nate will hear from colleges soon, and will graduate from high school in two months. Emma loves art and writing and is planning what she'll do this summer. David and I go to jazz clubs, and love to discover new musicians. My hair is growing back; last week I had my first bad hair day, and it was glorious! For spring break, the four of us are going to Sedona, Arizona, where we'll hike the red rocks together.

My cancer experience reminds me of the quote below from the great book, *The Hours,* by Michael Cunningham. Have you read it?

"Yes, Clarissa thinks, it's time for the day to be over. We throw our parties; we abandon our families to live alone in Canada; we struggle to write books that do not change the world, despite our gifts and our unstinting efforts, our most extravagant hopes. We live our lives, do whatever we do, and then we sleep—it's as simple and ordinary as that. A few jump out of windows or drown themselves or take pills; more die by accident; and most of us, the vast majority, are slowly devoured by some disease or, if we're very fortunate, by time itself. *There's just this for consolation: an hour here or there when our lives seem, against all odds and expectations, to burst open and give us everything we've ever imagined,* even though everyone but children (and perhaps even they) knows these hours will inevitably be followed by others, far darker and more difficult. Still, we cherish the city, the morning; we hope, more than anything, for more. Heaven only knows why we love it so."

Jen, I can't thank you enough for being my "gentle reader" through all of this. Parts of it were very scary, especially in the beginning, and it helped that no matter what was going on

I could write to you and I knew that you would read it, care, and respond. Once I had one dose of all the different kinds of chemo I wasn't so scared, and after the mid-chemo re-staging tests were OK I felt I could conquer the world. And you were always there, through all of it.

Being able to write to you about my cancer helped me for so many reasons. I got to express myself, to understand how I felt by writing about it, and to create something to leave behind even if I didn't make the 50/50 shot. Also, writing this book allowed me to feel that my cancer served a purpose: I produced something that might help others, either by offering suggestions on how to deal with cancer or by simply providing distraction during those long days of treatment and recovery. And I hope I can hold on to what I learned about savoring celebrations, even if the cancer is gone for good.

I wonder—what's next?

Love
Laura

Characters (in alphabetical order)

Cindy: Friend of Laura's. She is the Chief Technologist in Breast Imaging at the hospital where Laura works, and she and Laura have known each other for 17 years.

David: Laura's husband. When the book opens, Laura and David have been married for 24 years. David is a doctor specializing in Infectious Diseases, a native New Yorker who loves jazz, and an incredible husband and father.

Ellen: Author and former scientific consultant who wrote the book "Every Other Thursday" about a group of women who meet every two weeks to give each other mutual support and guidance. She encourages Laura to write about her cancer experience.

Emma: Laura's daughter. When the book opens she is 14, a freshman in high school. She is full of joy and has an innate sense of style. She loves art and writing.

Gerald: A physician-scientist at Memorial who makes discoveries in the lab and applies them to developing new, targeted anti-cancer drugs.

Jennifer: Friend of Laura's, to whom most of the emails in the book are directed. Jennifer and Laura met in a chamber music class in New York City ten years ago and keep in touch mostly by email. Jennifer is a child psychologist who lives with her husband and daughter in Philadelphia. She is also a fabulous cellist.

Jimmie: A psychiatrist and former Chair of the Department of Psychiatry at Laura's hospital.

Laura: A doctor at a cancer hospital who develops cancer. Laura is married to David and has two children, Nate and Emma.

Mark: Laura's brilliant and kind neurosurgeon, originally a boy from Tennessee who couldn't sing.

Maureen: Friend of Laura's, also a doctor at the cancer hospital where Laura works. Maureen has had cancer and fears nothing.

Mel: A breast surgeon in California, who has known Laura for years through meetings and publications.

Memorial Hospital/Memorial Sloan-Kettering Cancer Center, New York, NY: The finest cancer hospital in the world, where Laura has been a doctor and, at the beginning of the book, becomes a patient.

Mike: A breast pathologist in California who is a friend of Laura's. In his spare time, Mike participates in Triathlons. He is of Greek descent, an expert in ichthyology (the study of fish), and a friend and scientific collaborator of Mel's.

Monique (aka "Q"): Friend and neighbor of Laura and her family. She and Laura met in the park when their oldest children were babies and have been close ever since.

Nate: Laura's son. When the book opens he is 17, a high school junior applying to college. Nate likes community service, teaching, and writing.

Phil: Laura's oncologist, one of the best lymphoma doctors in the world. He saves lives.

Sam: Laura's neurologist, an expert in malignancies of the nervous system.

Terri: A doctor at Laura's hospital specializing in medical oncology. In addition to caring for patients, she creates film documentaries about cancer.

Glossary of Medical Terms

Anesthesia: Numbing medicine. Anesthesia can be local (at a specific site, either by injection, spray, or cream), with the patient awake, or general (administered intravenously or by inhalation), in which the patient is generally asleep and breathing is assisted by a respirator or ventilator (breathing machine).

Biopsy: Taking a sample of tissue with a needle or with surgery to send to the pathology laboratory so it can be examined under the microscope to determine if cancer is present.

Bone marrow: The site of development of blood cells, including red blood cells that carry oxygen in the blood, white blood cells that fight infection, and platelets that help the blood clot. In a bone marrow biopsy, a sample of bone marrow is removed, usually from the pelvis, to determine if malignant cells are present.

Catheter: A small tube that allows access to a particular part of the body. These may be placed through the skin.

Chemotherapy: Strong medication to kill cancer cells. Most chemotherapy works by killing rapidly dividing cells. Unfortunately, some normal cells divide rapidly, such as the cells in the bone marrow responsible for making blood cells.

Cerebrospinal fluid (CSF): The fluid surrounding the brain and spinal cord.

Cytology: Analysis of cells under the microscope.

Fingerstick: A method of obtaining blood for a blood test by sticking a small needle in a fingertip and obtaining a few drops of blood to put on a glass slide.

Intrathecal: Adjective: a route of administration for medication (such as chemotherapy) directly into the cerebrospinal fluid (CSF), the fluid around the brain and spinal cord. Intrathecal medication can be injected by performing a lumbar puncture (LP; also known as a spinal tap), a procedure in which a needle is inserted into the back to take fluid from around the spinal cord, or by using an Omaya, a sterile reservoir and tube that is implanted neurosurgically into the head.

Intravenous (IV): Adjective: a route of administration into a blood vessel (vein) of fluids, medication, or blood products. Noun: a small plastic tube placed into a vein (blood vessel) to administer the above items.

Leukovorin rescue: After administration of methotrexate, which is toxic chemotherapy, the leukovorin "rescue" involves repeated doses of an intravenous medication called leucovorin which helps combat the toxic effects of methotrexate.

Lumbar puncture (LP): a procedure in which a needle is inserted usually into the back between the third and fourth lumbar vertebrae (back bones) into the sac of fluid around the spinal cord to remove cerebrospinal fluid (CSF), the fluid around the spinal cord and brain. Synonym: spinal tap.

Lymph nodes: "Glands" containing lymphocytes, a type of white blood cell that participates in defending the body from infection. Lymph nodes can become enlarged in infections, inflammatory conditions, and malignant tumors.

Lymphocytes: A type of white blood cells that normally participate in defending the body from infection. There are different types of lymphocytes (B cells and T cells) with specialized immune functions. In autoimmune diseases, the lymphocytes attack the body as if it were foreign.

Lymphoma: A malignancy in which lymphocytes grow uncontrollably. Lymphoma can involve multiple body sites, including lymph nodes (the glands that swell up during infection), bone marrow (where new blood cells are produced), and other organs.

Magnetic resonance imaging (MRI): An imaging test applicable to any part of the body. MRI uses strong magnetic fields to make signals that are displayed as images.

Median survival: The amount of time for which half of the patients live less and half live more. A median survival of one year, for example, means that half of the patients live less than one year and half live more than one year.

Mediport: A type of catheter (sterile plastic tube) that can be placed into a vein under sterile conditions to allow access for intravenous medications. The tip of the tube is in the vein, and the port or reservoir that is injected is placed underneath the skin. To access the Mediport, the nurse or doctor must pierce the skin with a needle.

Methotrexate: A form of chemotherapy that attacks rapidly dividing cells.

Monoclonal antibody: A pure population of proteins that attack a specific target, such as a particular cell surface marker in the body. Monoclonal antibodies are an example of "targeted therapy," in which the treatment is specifically designed to attack a particular target, rather than to cause generalized death of rapidly dividing cells. Because monoclonal antibodies are more specific, they generally have fewer side effects than chemotherapy.

Nadir: In general parlance, "nadir" means the lowest point (opposite of zenith, the highest point). In medicine, "nadir" refers to having an extremely low count of white blood cells responsible for fighting infection in the body.

Neutropenia: Low count of neutrophils, a group of white blood cells that fight infection.

Neutrophil: A type of white blood cell, also called a polymorphonuclear leukocyte or "poly," that fights infection.

Omaya: A sterile tube that has its tip in the fluid around the brain (cerebrospinal fluid, or CSF). The Omaya must be placed neurosurgically by drilling a hole in the skull and inserting the catheter through brain tissue until it reaches one of the lateral ventricles, CSF-containing structures in the brain. Chemotherapy can be administered through the Omaya, and fluid can be removed from the Omaya ("Omaya tap") to determine if malignant cells are present.

pH: A quantitative measure of acidity. A fluid pH of 7.0 is "neutral," <7.0 is "acidic," and >7.0 is "alkaline" or "basic." Oral bicarbonate can make the urine more alkaline.

Port: The general term for a catheter (sterile plastic tube) placed into a vein to allow access for IV medications. A Mediport is a specific type of port.

Prednisone: An oral steroid that can be used to treat a variety of diseases, including lymphomas. Prednisone can cause weight gain, sleep disturbances, and manic episodes.

R-CHOP: An intravenous chemotherapy regimen used to treat some lymphomas. R is Rituximab, a monoclonal antibody directed against specific malignant B lymphocytes; C is cyclophosphamide; H is doxorubicin; O is vincristine (originally called Oncovin); and P is prednisone, an oral steroid.

Remission: Control of active malignancy. Patients in remission may stay healthy or may redevelop malignancy in the future ("recurrence").

Stage IV: Disseminated malignancy. This is the most advanced stage of cancer, when sites other than the location of the index tumor are involved, and has the worst outcome.

Targeted therapy: Anti-cancer treatment that specifically attacks malignant cells, without significant damage to normal cells. Hopefully, this approach will become available for many cancers, providing effective therapy with minimal side effects.

Ventricles of the brain: Four fluid-filled structures in the brain that contain cerebrospinal fluid (CSF) and communicate with the CSF around the brain and spinal cord. The brain has two lateral ventricles (one on the right and one on the left) and two midline ventricles (the third and the fourth).